"Tina Ruggiero clearly understands that nutrition and great taste can happily coexist. She is the voice of reason when it comes to modern nutrition science, and her recipes are as smart as they are delicious, creative and accessible. Tina has given us a wonderful gift with this book; it's a must-have in every kitchen!"

—Josie Bissett, award-winning actress, author, model and mother of two

"In *The Truly Healthy Family Cookbook*, award-winning nutrition expert Tina Ruggiero delivers what we all crave: an approachable cookbook filled with inventive, playful recipes that pack a powerful nutrient punch. From her Homemade Müesli to her kale and pumpkin seed Power Pesto to simple desserts like Strawberries on a Cloud, Ruggiero proves that healthful eating can be fun, decadent and satisfying, without a huge amount of effort."

—Cheryl Sternman Rule, author of *Ripe: A Fresh, Colorful Approach to Fruits and Vegetables*

"Eating healthy is critical, and Tina provides us with fresh, innovative recipes, tips and techniques for wholesome cooking. Tina's simple, delicious and family-friendly meals use readily available ingredients and empower us to make meals we can feel good about serving our loved ones. This book enriches our fast-paced daily lives and inspires each of us to be confident when preparing super-nutritious meals, snacks and beverages."

—Qian Yuan, M.D., PhD, FAAP, Harvard Medical School

"As dietitians, we're thrilled that Tina's recipes are super healthy, but as foodies we applaud the fact that they're tasty, too. Teaching families how to enjoy a wholesome and delicious diet is a top priority for us; *The Truly Healthy Family Cookbook* is definitely moving to the top of our recommended cookbook list."

—Janice Newell Bissex M.S., R.D. and Liz Weiss, M.S., R.D., founders of MealMakeoverMoms.com, authors, *NO WHINE WITH DINNER: 150 Healthy, Kid-Tested Recipes from The Meal Makeover Moms*

"Healthy and flavorful—if you're still wondering how to convince your family that good-for-you can taste marvelous, pick up this book. Tina Ruggiero's enthusiasm is contagious. She will surprise you over and over again with her fresh and innovative recipes. Best of all, her book also showcases ancient grains and flours—from quinoa and brown rice, to buckwheat and amaranth. What's not to like?"

—Maria Speck, author of *Ancient Grains for Modern Meals, a New York Times* notable book and winner of the Julia Child Award

"Tina is all about no-nonsense nutrition. Her recipes are superfood stars; her insight will make you smarter and healthier, and her book is motivational. You'll want to get in the kitchen, fire up your stove and make simply amazing meals for the ones you love."

—Jennifer Cohen, bestselling author, Certified Personal Trainer on *Shedding for the Wedding*

"When it comes to eating right, or perhaps more important, cooking right, my go-to person has always been Tina. With my schedule and all the dangerously tempting food options out there, that's a clearcut recipe for disaster, but Tina always goes back to the basics, and then provides the answers to keep me—and just about everyone else—on the right track. Nothing beats common sense backed with facts and good judgment, and that clearly defines Tina's advice."

—Peter Greenberg, CBS NEWS

"Being a chef, I believe that what you put into a dish is what you get out of it. Tina brings this tenant to life, with her simple approach to wholesome cooking; she streamlines recipes to get the most nutrition and taste from meals while using only the best ingredients that will deliver health and wellbeing. *The Truly Healthy Family Cookbook* is an essential addition to any home cook's library."

—Executive Chef Brandon McGlamery, Luma on *Park & Prato Winter Park*

"Tina Ruggiero embodies what every nutrition expert should be: She bases her counsel on sound science; she has a passion for food and the skills to create mouth-watering recipes that are tempting and healthy, and she looks and acts the part by living her philosophy to her very core."

—Tara Gidus, M.S., R.D., author of *Pregnancy Cooking & Nutrition for Dummies*

"Tina leads the way for those seeking more nutrition and enjoyment from the foods they eat. Her new book is packed with simple yet irresistible recipes you won't find in any other family cookbook. Accurate nutrition information separates fact from fiction; beautiful photos illustrate her recipes, and Tina's cooking tips will make anyone a confident, healthy cook in no time."

—Chef Harry, The Colt Culinary Project, author, Host of *Chef Harry & Friends*

"If you find yourself running short on time and only making your family quick fix meals that leave you feeling guilty, this book is for you. The recipes in *The Truly Healthy Family Cookbook* are a triple threat—simple, mega-nutritious and super-tasty. Make it your go-to resource and you will never have to stress about what's for breakfast, lunch or dinner again!"

—Liza Utter, Entertaining & Hosting expert, Founder, Life's a Party Inc.

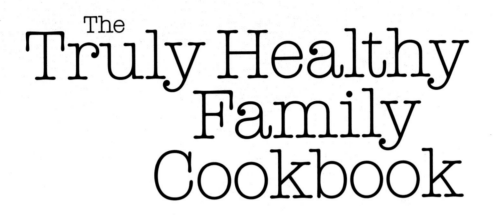

The
Truly Healthy
Family
Cookbook

The Truly Healthy Family Cookbook

BASED ON CUTTING-EDGE NUTRITION SCIENCE

Mega-nutritious Meals that are Inspired, Delicious and Fad-free

TINA RUGGIERO, M.S., R.D.

NATIONAL SPEAKER ON NUTRITION, TV PERSONALITY,
HEALTH COLUMNIST AND BESTSELLING AUTHOR

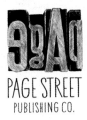

PAGE STREET
PUBLISHING CO.

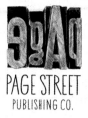

PAGE STREET
PUBLISHING CO.

First published in 2013 by
Page Street Publishing
27 Congress Street, Suite 205-10
Salem, MA 01970
www.pagestreetpublishing.com

Distributed by Macmillan; sales in Canada by The Canadian Manda Group; distribution in Canada by The Jaguar Book Group.

16   15   14   13   1   2   3   4   5

ISBN-13: 978-1-62414-008-2
ISBN-10: 1-62414-008-4

Library of Congress Control Number: 2013933895

Cover and book design by Page Street Publishing
Photography by Bill Bettencourt
Food Stylist: Brandon Bills

Printed and bound in China

For my mother,
my angel,
without whom this book
would not be a reality

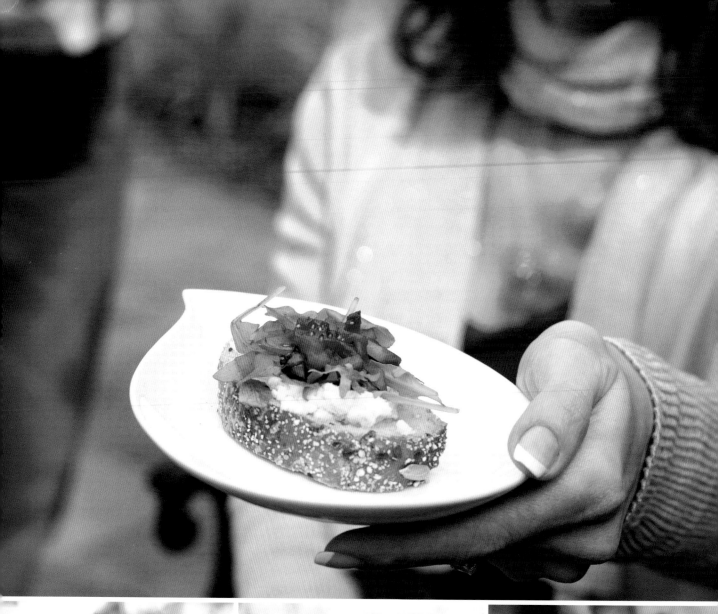

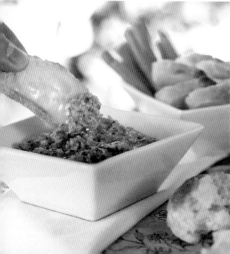

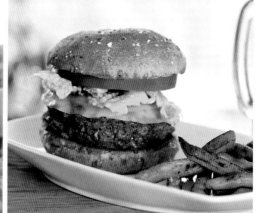

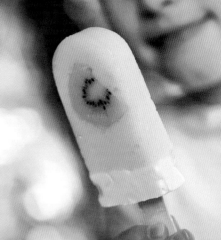

Contents

FOREWORD 11

INTRODUCTION 14

Better Breakfasts and Brunch 17
OUT WITH THE OLD, IN WITH THE NEW! THESE BOLD-FLAVOR OPTIONS REV UP
YOUR REPERTOIRE AND KEEP YOU ENERGIZED.

Easy-Peasy Panini and Sandwiches 45
FILL UP, NOT OUT, WITH THESE SCRUMPTIOUS LUNCHES!

Power Proteins from Land and Sea 63
MORE FLAVOR, FEWER CALORIES, BETTER HEALTH. BRING IT!

Tempting Pasta, Flatbread and One-Dish Wonders 91
SIMPLE, FILLING RECIPES THAT WILL SATISFY THE BIGGEST APPETITES
WHILE KEEPING CALORIES IN CHECK!

Simply Sensational Salad Meals and Side Dishes 115
GIVE MEALTIME A MAKEOVER WITH EXCITING RECIPES THAT DELIVER
HEALTH AND DELICIOUSNESS!

Sweet Surprises 141
SAVE ROOM FOR DESSERT! GUILT-FREE TREATS MAKE HAPPY ENDINGS!

Supercharged Snacks and Nibbles 159
WHETHER IT'S MIDDAY OR MIDNIGHT, THESE SWEET AND SAVORY MUNCHIES
OFFER SATISFACTION AND NUTRITION!

Luscious Libations 183
PERK UP YOUR DAYS AND NIGHTS WITH HEALTHY COFFEES, TEAS AND SKINNY COCKTAILS!

REFERENCES 200

ACKNOWLEDGMENTS 205

RECIPE INDEX 206

INDEX 208

ABOUT THE AUTHOR 223

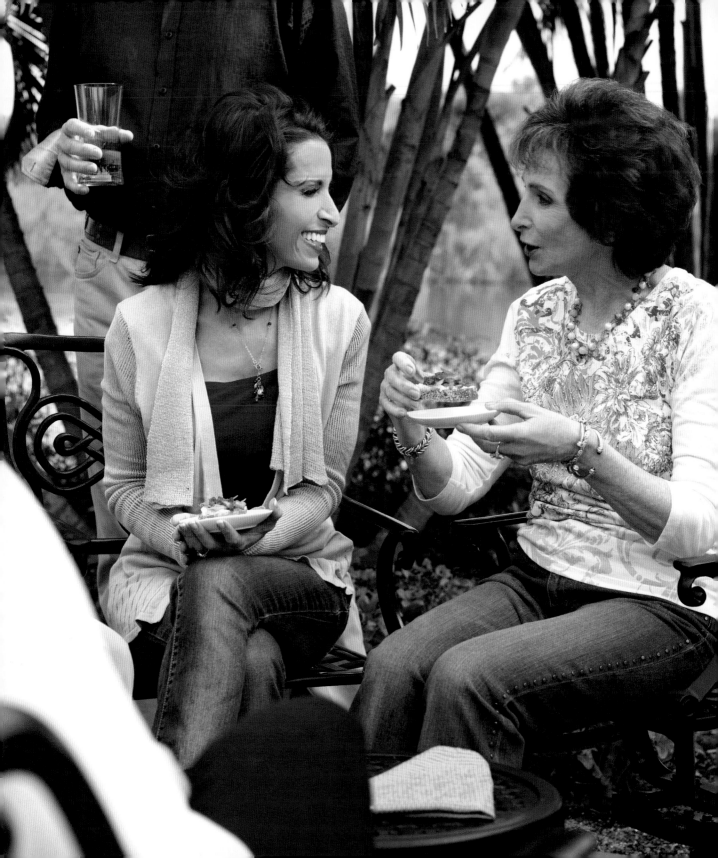

Foreword

EATING AND COOKING ARE CHERISHED AND SACRED RITUALS OF DAILY LIFE. We congregate, we share, we nurture, we plan and we love around meals. No doubt, we all celebrate our food. But the content of food, like the content of the rest of our life activities—whether it be work, play or exercise—is so important to our health and well-being. Let's face it—delicious, nutritious food is a critical part of living well. It is a cornerstone of our overall wellness and health.

In spite of the abundance of healthy food options, getting people to cook and eat healthfully is not easy. For one, we now rarely cook and eat at home. The age-old pastime of the home-cooked meal is fast becoming an anachronism. As a kid growing up in the 1960s, my family rarely ate out. Today, Americans dine out five times a week.

The lower price of food and the greater accessibility to the supply of food sources have led to this "fast" food revolution. Demands of modern lifestyles—longer work hours, single-parent households and two working-parent households—also make the challenge of cooking at home more daunting and processed foods more appealing. But this is why nutritional and culinary education should become a necessary part of modern-day life.

Besides obesity, poor diet is a primary cause of a number of chronic diseases. Poor dietary habits—the most notable of which are excessive salt, fat and calorie consumption—are inter-related risk factors for the most common yet difficult to treat diseases. Dietary factors are also associated with various cancers, and inadequate nutrition, low dietary calcium and vitamin D are causes for osteoporosis.

As a physician, I know how difficult it can be to get people to adopt healthy behaviors. But healthy eating and cooking, like exercising, is much easier when you use an informed, motivated approach. This is what attracted me to *The Truly Healthy Family Cookbook.* Tina uses a basic, no-fad and matter-of-fact approach to cooking and nutrition. Starting with the premise that we need to eat healthfully and enjoy it, she has created a well-rounded fund of recipes that draw from many regions of food origin, food types and palates.

When you read this book, you won't feel overwhelmed by the task of cooking a meal or paralyzed by an avalanche of nutrition information. Healthy cooking here is accessible, practical, mouthwatering and simply appealing. The content of each recipe is fully explained, so there is no mystery involved about nutrition or taste. Every ingredient has a purpose. Every recipe has value. Every recipe has an omnipotent role in the diet.

Needless to say, Tina's recipes are as easy to digest as the end product itself. The difference between this cookbook and others I've seen is that *The Truly Healthy Family Cookbook* presents an informed approach to eating that emphasizes not just nutrition but also its connection to basic, varied and flavorful ingredients. Her reassuring tone is balanced, informed, savory and fun, making healthy cooking and eating accessible to even the novice.

The nutrition and food worlds have been inundated with "new" methodology and unqualified "experts" who have fostered confusion about the real issues and the basics of nutrition, but Tina is to be believed. Her impressive credentials, her decades of practical experience, her talent as a cook and her nature to nurture body and mind culminate in a book that should be in everyone's kitchen. *The Truly Healthy Family Cookbook* is relevant to families large and small; you don't even need to have children to reap long-lasting benefits from this book. It upholds the values of family meals—inviting, fresh, nutritionally sound and absolutely delicious.

Alex C. Simotas, M.D.
Assistant Professor and Attending Physician
Department of Physiatry
Hospital for Special Surgery
Weill Cornell Medical College

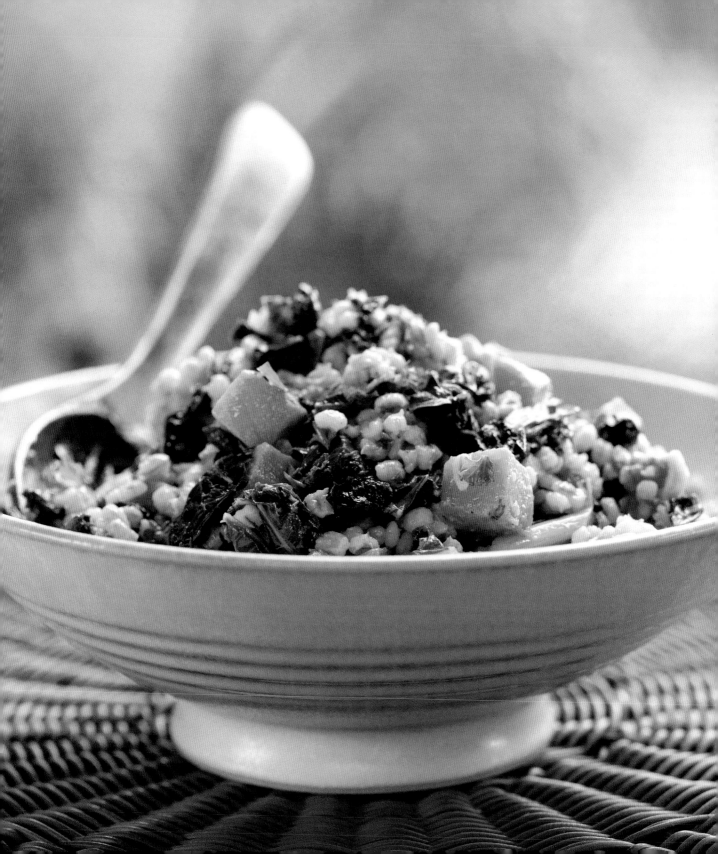

Introduction

I like to keep things simple.

I've been known to write my recipes in pencil on a notepad. Maybe it's the smell of lead or the crinkling sound the paper makes when I turn the page, but there's something soothing about the tangibility of creating. I think that's why I like to cook. And it should come as no surprise that I prefer cookbooks to tablet computers. I can write in the margins, making notes about ingredients or adjustments, and the occasional smudge of butter on the page is like my personal stamp: *Tina was here!*

When it comes to food, I also lean toward the traditional. I like pasta made from semolina flour. I like roasted chestnuts come holiday time, and nothing beats a glass of cold milk with one of my homemade dark chocolate walnut brownies. I love to barbecue, and I don't plan to give up cheese anytime soon. It's a staple in my home along with bread and eggs.

To be honest, I'm not sure when eating became so complex. To eat well these days, you're made to feel as if you need degrees in biochemistry, economics and maybe political science. Self-purported "experts" with an agenda make you feel compelled to buy this ingredient or that, or boycott this product or that one. Well, I don't have an agenda. I just love good food and the quality of life and well-being it allows. So, I wrote this cookbook for those of you like me: you believe in delicious, fresh food made from scratch, smart ingredients, small portions and simple preparation.

I love to cook and eat all types of foods—I believe in bold taste and instant gratification—but I do so with health, simplicity and enjoyment at the forefront of my mind. Every one of my recipes features ingredients that contribute valuable nutrition to your diet. I mix herbs with vegetables and fruits with dairy, creating powerful meals that pack a wallop of vitamins and minerals into sensible portions. And that's what makes this cookbook different from what you'll find elsewhere. I've created healthy recipes using meats, cheeses, wheat and nuts, allowing your family to enjoy their favorite foods without compromising nutrition or taste.

Plus, each recipe uses readily available ingredients and doesn't require special skills or lots of time to prepare. Honestly, when you finish cooking from this book, I want you to feel like a modern-day Wonder Woman or Superman in the kitchen. I don't incorporate molecular cuisine, so you won't be making colloids here, and I won't tell you to avoid everything but vegetables and eat them raw. This book is about keeping it real, and what it aspires to be is your go-to reference for delicious, healthy, everyday food.

I've never been a fan of fad diets and food substitutions, so if you're looking for recipes that use turkey to make meatloaf or pita bread to make nacho chips, this isn't the book for you. But if you're looking for simple recipes that use your favorite foods (plus some new, soon-to-be favorites) to broaden your repertoire, add nutrition to meals, satisfy your family and tempt your taste buds, then you're in for a treat.

Each recipe will add to your regular rotation of meals, so don't be afraid of what may seem different. Open the door to new ingredients and explore their possibilities. Your reward is discovering inspired flavors, delicious dishes and things you never thought you could do yourself! This book will empower you in the kitchen, instill confidence and a deeper understanding of nutrition and make every meal enjoyable, not to mention healthier. You'll also find that each recipe introduces you to cooking methods, tips or techniques that will improve your skills in the kitchen. I believe that a confident cook is a good one.

Being healthy is a conscious choice you make, and health can be achieved by eating all foods. Is this easy? No. Temptation lurks around every corner. Healthy cooking and living takes thought, effort, application and dedication, but repetition is the mother of habit. So, my wish for you is that you sink into healthy eating habits as you would a warm blanket. Cook your way through this book, write in the margins, try what you wouldn't otherwise and apply my philosophy of enjoying everything in small, tasty, healthy portions. You will not be disappointed.

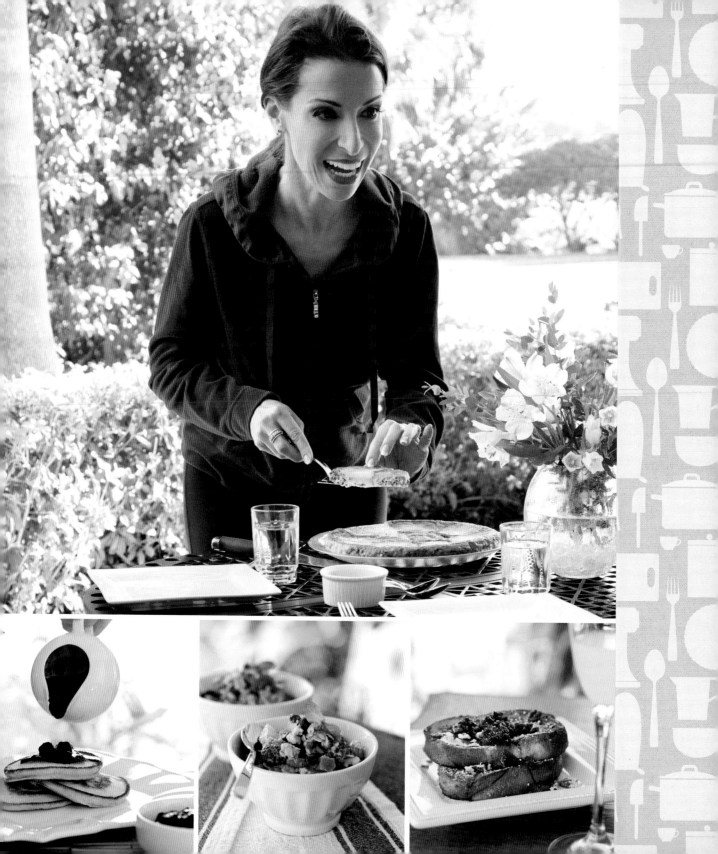

Better Breakfasts and Brunch

Out with the old, in with the new! These bold-flavor options rev up your repertoire and keep you energized.

Tutti Frutti, Sunday Special, Mix It Up Müesli and All-Star Kale and Potato Frittata—these are the reasons my family eats breakfast. The options may not be traditional, but they're healthy and delicious, and that's why everyone finds a place around the kitchen table each and every morning.

Let's face it—basic breakfast food can get boring. Especially when you're in a rush or don't have much of an appetite, there's no incentive to eat this all-important meal, but breakfast really does live up to its reputation!

Breakfast eaters find it easier to stay slim and have more energy and improved productivity. Breakfast can also boost your mood and, in younger children, breakfast can give a competitive edge, reduce hyperactivity, increase concentration and improve performance.

However, eating just anything in the morning is not much better than skipping breakfast. Sugary or high-fat foods will actually slow you down, and this is another reason some people don't care for breakfast; they feel sluggish after eating. What to do? Focus on nutrients and not necessarily the food. There's no rule that says we have to eat cereal in the morning.

To energize your body and boost brainpower, think outside the cereal box. A healthy breakfast includes some protein, which can come from fish, eggs, cheese or quinoa. You'll need some fiber, which can come from nuts, colorful fruits or veggies. A little bit of fat will prevent you from craving mid-morning snacks, and you'll want to include some complex carbohydrates from grains such as couscous, oats or bulgur to keep your metabolism humming.

By approaching breakfast with this philosophy, your options become endlessly more tempting!

Mix It Up MÜESLI

HOMEMADE MÜESLI WITH OATS, ALMOND MILK, KEFIR AND FRUIT

Nothing compares to the taste and nutrition of homemade müesli, and what you buy in the store (resembling granola) is a far cry from the original recipe. Authentic müesli is made with raw oats, which contain phytic acid, a nutrient that may help protect us from cancer. In fact, every ingredient in this recipe contributes to good health. Also, it's quick and easy to make, and you can adapt the recipe to your taste preferences, the season or whatever you have on hand. Each serving is rich in complex carbohydrates, fiber and calcium, and just one serving of müesli can provide two servings of fruit.

YIELD: 6 cups | **TIME:** 20 minutes

4 oz/120 ml almond milk, unsweetened

2 cups/475 ml vanilla kefir

1 ¼ cups/100 g oats, rolled, old-fashioned

½ medium apple, peeled and grated

¼ cup/40 g grapes, halved

½ cup/75 g raisins

¼ cup/40 g pecans, chopped and toasted

6 oz/180 g nonfat Greek yogurt

¼ cup/60 ml honey

2 tbsp/30 ml lemon juice

Mint leaves, for garnish (optional)

Combine all the ingredients but the mint in a large bowl. Cover and store in the refrigerator for a minimum of 24 hours. When ready to serve, ladle into bowls and garnish with mint. Will last 3 days tightly covered in the refrigerator.

PER 1-CUP SERVING: Calories 280, protein 9 g, total fat 7 g, carbohydrates 45 g, sodium 65 mg, fiber 3 g

TINA'S TIP: Feel free to experiment and make this recipe your own. Try adding apricots, ground flaxseed or wheat germ; use walnuts or hazelnuts instead of pecans; and top it with sliced bananas, strawberries or raspberries.

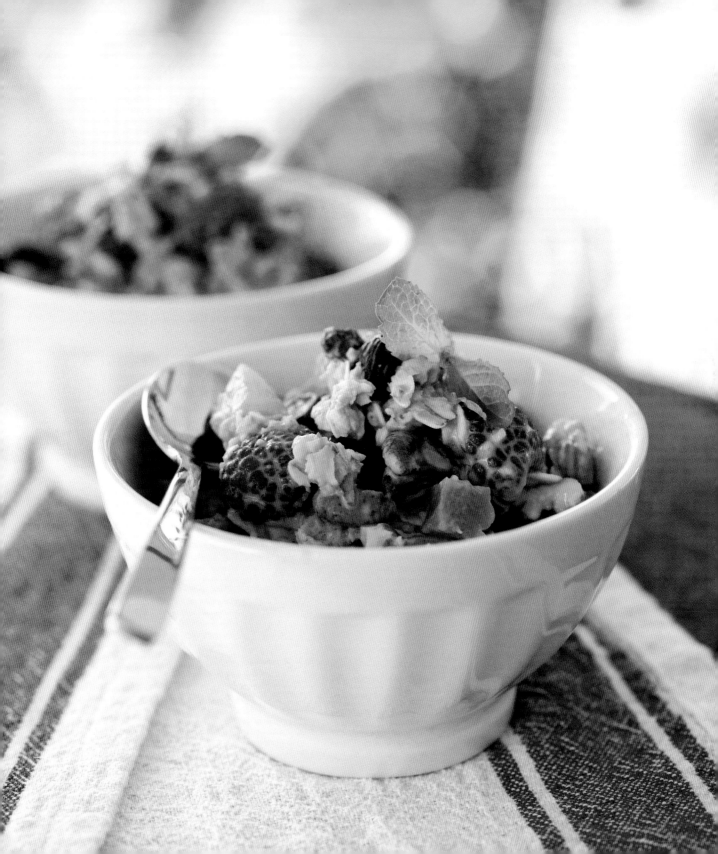

Flip for **FLAPJACKS**

MULTIGRAIN PANCAKES WITH APPLE-ORANGE-HONEY TOPPING

Every ingredient in this recipe has a nutritional benefit, but all my family knows is that a stack of these pancakes are the perfect start to a Sunday morning! I've also been known to make these for the occasional dinner. No matter when you enjoy these pancakes, you'll love the taste. They're a little different than traditional pancakes, but that's what makes them a winner in my home. My secret ingredient is buttermilk. Packing more calcium and protein than regular milk, buttermilk is also a rich source of gut-healthy probiotics. Yogurt is not your only source! Also, if you have a few different types of flour in your cupboard, you can make this recipe with a number of options (see tip). Otherwise, the fragrant spices, hearty oats and naturally-sweet fruit in this recipe will inspire you to toss the packaged pancake mixes and convert to scratch. You'll never go back!

YIELD: 16 pancakes | **TIME:** 30 minutes

---

2 Granny Smith apples, peeled, cored and grated

Zest (2 tsp/8 g) and juice of 2 oranges (½ cup/120 ml)

1 cup/235 ml honey

¾ cup/90 g all-purpose flour

½ cup/60 g whole wheat flour

1 cup/56 g wheat germ

1 cup/80 g quick-cooking oats

1 tsp/2.3 g cinnamon

¼ tsp nutmeg

2 ¼ tsp/10.4 g baking powder

½ tsp baking soda

½ tsp salt

2 cups/470 ml low-fat buttermilk

2 eggs

1 tsp/5 ml vanilla extract

Vegetable oil, for cooking

To make the topping, place the grated apple, zest and juice of the oranges and the honey in a small saucepan. Bring to a simmer and cook until the apples are translucent and the mixture has thickened to a spoonable sauce, about 20 minutes. Yield should be about 2 cups/475 milliliters.

While the topping is cooking, prepare the pancakes. Preheat oven to 200°F/ 93°C. In a large bowl combine the all-purpose flour, whole wheat flour, wheat germ, oats, cinnamon, nutmeg, baking powder, baking soda and salt. Whisk to combine.

In a medium bowl, whisk together the buttermilk, eggs and vanilla. Stir them into the dry ingredients just to combine. Do not overmix. Mixture will be somewhat thick.

Heat a nonstick skillet over medium heat. Brush the pan with a small amount of vegetable oil. For each pancake, scoop a heaping ¼ cup/60 milliliters batter onto the skillet. Pancakes should be approximately 4 inches/10 centimeters across. Cook the pancakes for 2 to 3 minutes on the first side, or until golden brown. Flip the pancakes and cook another 2 to 3 minutes. Place pancakes in the oven for up to 10 minutes to keep warm if needed.

PER PANCAKE: Calories 150, protein 6 g, total fat 2 g, carbohydrates 28 g, sodium 290 mg, fiber 3 g

TINA'S TIP: Try using different flours like quinoa or amaranth flour or adding nuts or dried fruits to the mix. Substitute quinoa and amaranth one-for-one for whole wheat, but dont use them for the entire amount—they are too grainy and don't have enough gluten.

Tutti **FRUITTI**

MIXED FRESH FRUIT SALAD WITH CINNAMON-RAISIN CROUTONS

The Tuscan region of Italy brought us the much-loved panzanella salad, a simple dish made with chunks of bread and fresh tomatoes. It's so simple to make yet incredibly delicious – and it happens to be the inspiration for this fruit salad! Who says croutons and fruit can't go together, especially when the croutons are made with whole wheat, cinnamon-raisin bread? Yum! Dusted with cinnamon, the croutons get a boost of nutrition, and you'll benefit from the spice's anti-bacterial powers and its ability to stabilize blood pressure. Further, my fruit mix is a treasure trove of health: kiwi has more vitamin C than an orange; strawberries fight cancer, blueberries protect our vision and grapes combat heart disease.

YIELD: 8 servings | **TIME:** 25 minutes

4 slices whole wheat cinnamon-raisin bread, cut into bite-size pieces

¾ tsp ground cinnamon

2 tsp/4 g sugar

1 tbsp/15 ml canola oil

1 tbsp/15 ml honey

1 tbsp/15 ml lemon juice

1 cup/145 g blueberries

2 cups/300 g grapes, halved

1 ½ cups/255 g sliced strawberries

4 kiwis, chopped

Preheat oven to 325°F/170°C or gas mark 3.

Line a rimmed baking sheet with foil. Add the diced bread pieces. In a small bowl, combine the cinnamon, sugar and canola oil. Toss the bread with the cinnamon mixture to coat. Bake until golden and crispy, 15 to 20 minutes. Remove from the oven and let cool.

Meanwhile, in a large bowl, add the honey and lemon juice, mixing to combine. Add the blueberries, grapes, strawberries and kiwi, tossing to combine everything. When ready to serve, combine the fruit with the croutons.

PER SERVING: Calories 140, protein 3 g, total fat 4 g, carbohydrates 27 g, sodium 75 mg, fiber 3 g

TINA'S TIP: Resist the temptation to increase the oven temperature higher than 325°F/170°C or gas mark 3. Yes, the croutons will crisp quicker, but they'll have a greater potential to burn. So, let them take their time browning while you chop up the fruit for the salad.

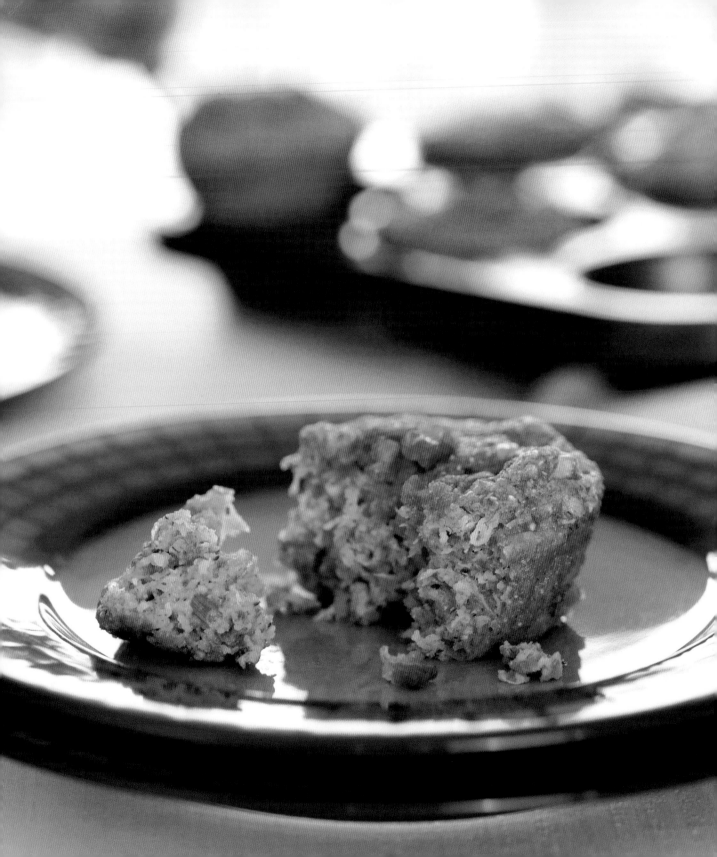

Little Miss
SAVORY MUFFINS

ZUCCHINI, SWEET POTATO, CHEDDAR AND PROSCIUTTO MUFFINS

Benefits of the Mediterranean diet are well known, and this muffin recipe combines many of the staples of this healthy way of eating, including whole grains, olive oil, vegetables and yogurt. Young and old alike find these muffins irresistible. They're the perfect size for little fingers and complement eggs and omelets. You can make them ahead of time, too, so sleeping in on Sunday morning is definitely an option! Just pop them into the oven to warm, and wait for the aroma to lure everyone into the kitchen. Leftovers? Enjoy them as an accompaniment to a salad or bowl of hearty soup.

YIELD: 12 muffins   **TIME:** 1 hour 15 minutes

---

1 cup/120 g whole wheat flour

½ cup/60 g buckwheat flour

½ cup/60 g all-purpose flour

1 tsp/5 g baking soda

¼ tsp baking powder

¼ tsp salt

6 tbsp/90 ml olive oil

4 ½ tbsp/67.5 g low-fat Greek yogurt

3 eggs

1 ½ cups/165 g shredded zucchini

1 ½ cups/165 g shredded sweet potato

1 tsp/15 g fresh thyme leaves

2 oz/58 g thinly sliced scallions

1 cup/120 g grated sharp Cheddar

½ cup/40 g finely chopped prosciutto

Preheat oven to 400°F/200°C or gas mark 6. Line a 12-cup muffin pan with paper liners.

Place the whole wheat flour, buckwheat flour, all-purpose flour, baking soda, baking powder and salt in a large bowl. Whisk together.

In another bowl, whisk the olive oil, yogurt and eggs together. Add the dry ingredients in a couple of batches, stirring to combine with a rubber spatula or wooden spoon. Do not overmix. Stir in the zucchini, sweet potato, thyme, scallions, Cheddar and half the prosciutto. Fill the muffin cups. Divide the remaining prosciutto among the muffins, sprinkling it on top and lightly pressing it into the batter. Bake for 45 minutes, or until a toothpick inserted into the center comes out clean.

PER MUFFIN: Calories 100, protein 4 g, total fat 5 g, carbohydrates 9 g, sodium 300, fiber 1 g

TINA'S TIP: Instead of prosciutto, try using smoked salmon. Serve with a little low-fat sour cream.

Rev Up 'n' Go
BAKED EGGS

BAKED EGGS WITH TOMATOES, SPINACH AND FONTINA CHEESE

Nothing is better than waking up to the smell of something yummy in the oven, and these baked eggs are no exception. They have the power to lure sleepyheads from their bedrooms to the kitchen! Quick and simple to make, these baked eggs are like little omelets in a cup, and they're just as delicious as they are healthy. One serving delivers 35 percent of a day's worth of vitamin A and 20 percent of your vitamin C requirement, and this one-dish meal is a very good source of quality protein. Nutmeg, my secret ingredient, is the perfect complement to the fontina cheese, and it contains eugenol, a powerful, fat-soluble antioxidant that's important for heart health. In my home, we enjoy these baked eggs nearly every Saturday morning, and to keep it fresh, I change the ingredients with the season.

YIELD: 4 servings | **TIME:** 25 minutes

Special equipment: 4 (6 to 8 oz/180 to 240 ml) ramekins or custard cups

1 tsp/5 ml vegetable oil

4 tbsp/40 g finely chopped shallot

4 oz/120 g roughly chopped spinach leaves

1 cup/240 g finely chopped tomato

¼ tsp salt

¼ tsp pepper

Several grates of nutmeg

4 eggs

¼ cup/60 ml cream

2 oz/60 g fontina cheese, grated

Preheat oven to 400°F/200°C or gas mark 6. Heat a small sauté pan over medium heat. Add the vegetable oil to the pan and sauté the shallot with a pinch of salt until softened but not brown, about 2 minutes. Add the spinach and wilt, then stir in the tomato. Season with the salt, pepper and nutmeg. Divide the mixture among the ramekins. Break an egg into each ramekin. Pour 1 tablespoon/20 milliliters of cream over each egg and sprinkle with a pinch of salt and a grating of black pepper. Divide the cheese among the ramekins. Bake for 10 minutes, or until the white is set and the yolk is still runny (or cook longer if a solid yolk is preferred). The cheese should be melted and starting to brown.

PER SERVING: Calories 220, protein 11 g, total fat 16 g, carbohydrates 9 g, sodium 320 mg, fiber 2 g

TINA'S TIP: Experiment with different fillings for variety. Kale can be used in place of spinach in the above version, and Serrano ham, onions and potatoes are also excellent variations. You really can't go wrong.

Superberry **SMOOTHIE**

RASPBERRY, PEACH, YOGURT, HONEY AND WHEAT GERM SMOOTHIE

This jewel-tone smoothie is as pretty as it is healthy! It contains raspberry ketones, which may inhibit the growth of cancer cells, and it's also rich in flavonoids, which may help fight heart disease. A dash of honey naturally sweetens this refreshing energizer, and my secret ingredient is wheat germ! It adds a slightly nutty flavor, but it's a powerhouse of nutrients: it's an excellent source of fiber and rich in vitamin E, folate, magnesium and omega-3 fatty acids. Buy a big jar of wheat germ and keep it in the refrigerator to maintain its freshness. Then, use it in muffins, protein shakes, quick breads, oatmeal, cereal and even casseroles!

YIELD: 1 smoothie (about 10 oz/300 ml) | **TIME:** 5 minutes

¾ cup/95 g raspberries

½ peach, roughly chopped

½ cup/120 g nonfat plain Greek yogurt

1 tsp/2.3 g wheat germ

1 tsp/5 ml honey

3 ice cubes

Place all ingredients in a blender and purée. The mixture will be thick, so pause the blender, scrape down the sides and purée again. Do this 2 or 3 times, or until it is smooth yet thick.

PER SERVING: Calories 100, protein 2 g, total fat 0.5 g, carbohydrates 27 g, sodium 0 mg, fiber 2 g

TINA'S TIP: For variety, this recipe is also delicious made with almond milk in place of the yogurt. Just omit the ice cubes and prepare the recipe as written.

Kiss My **CAKES**

CORNCAKES WITH BLUEBERRY COMPOTE

I know what you're thinking. "Corn? What's that doing in a healthy cookbook?" The answer is simple. Corn – especially cornmeal – is one of the few foods that are a source of lutein and zeaxanthin, two nutrients that are hugely important to prevent macular degeneration, for which there is no cure. Made with all-natural ingredients, these cakes contribute important nutrients to the diet and are an early morning crowd pleaser. Their texture is slightly different from pancakes, but if you like cornbread, cornbread muffins or cornbread stuffing, you'll enjoy these variations on the traditional flapjack. With virtually no fat and a super fruit topping, you'll feel good about putting this meal on the table. If you have leftover compote, use it to top waffles, toast or frozen yogurt!

YIELD: 5 servings (10 corncakes) | **TIME:** 40 minutes

1 ½ cups/225 g blueberries, thawed if frozen

½ cup/100 g sugar

½ tsp lemon zest

2 tbsp/30 ml lemon juice

1 ½ tsp/12 g cornstarch

¾ cup/105 g cornmeal

¼ cup/30 g whole wheat flour

¼ cup/30 g all-purpose flour

½ tsp baking powder

½ tsp baking soda

½ tsp salt

1 cup/235 ml buttermilk

2 eggs, beaten

2 tbsp/30 ml honey

1 to 2 tbsp/14 to 28 g unsalted butter, melted, for cooking

To make the compote, place the blueberries in a saucepan with the sugar and lemon zest. If using fresh berries add ½ cup/120 milliliters water. If frozen, the natural juices from thawing will provide enough liquid. Bring to a simmer and cook for about 10 minutes, until most of the berries have burst and the juices have cooked down and concentrated. While the berries are cooking, combine the lemon juice and cornstarch. Stir into the simmering berries. Cook an additional 2 minutes to thicken. Reserve. Compote can be made ahead and kept refrigerated for 2 weeks. Reheat before serving.

To make the corncakes, in a medium bowl, whisk together the cornmeal, whole wheat flour, all-purpose flour, baking powder, baking soda and salt. In a small bowl, whisk together the buttermilk, eggs and honey. Whisk the buttermilk mixture into the dry ingredients. Stir until just combined.

Preheat oven to 200°F/93°C. Heat a large nonstick skillet over medium-low heat. Brush with a small amount of butter. For each corncake, scoop ¼ cup/60 milliliters batter onto skillet. Cook until edges start to dry and lightly brown and bubbles form on the surface, about 2 minutes. Flip and continue to cook another minute until cooked through. Transfer to a baking tray. Continue until batter is used up. Place tray in the oven to warm pancakes briefly.

For each serving, place 2 pancakes on a plate and top with 2 tablespoons/30 milliliters of reserved compote.

PER PANCAKE: Calories 100, protein 4 g, total fat 2.5 g, carbohydrates 16 g, sodium 390 mg, fiber 1 g

PER 1 TABLESPOON/15 MILLILITERS COMPOTE: Calories 30, protein 0 g, total fat 0 g, carbohydrates 8 g, sodium 0 g, fiber 0 g

TINA'S TIP: For added texture, try adding corn kernels or quick-cooking oats to the batter.

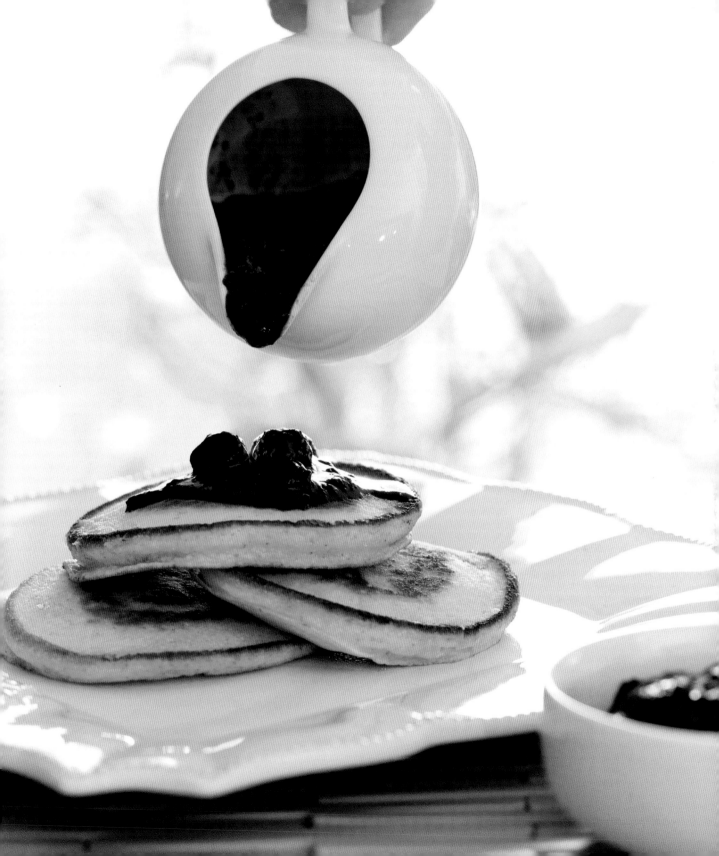

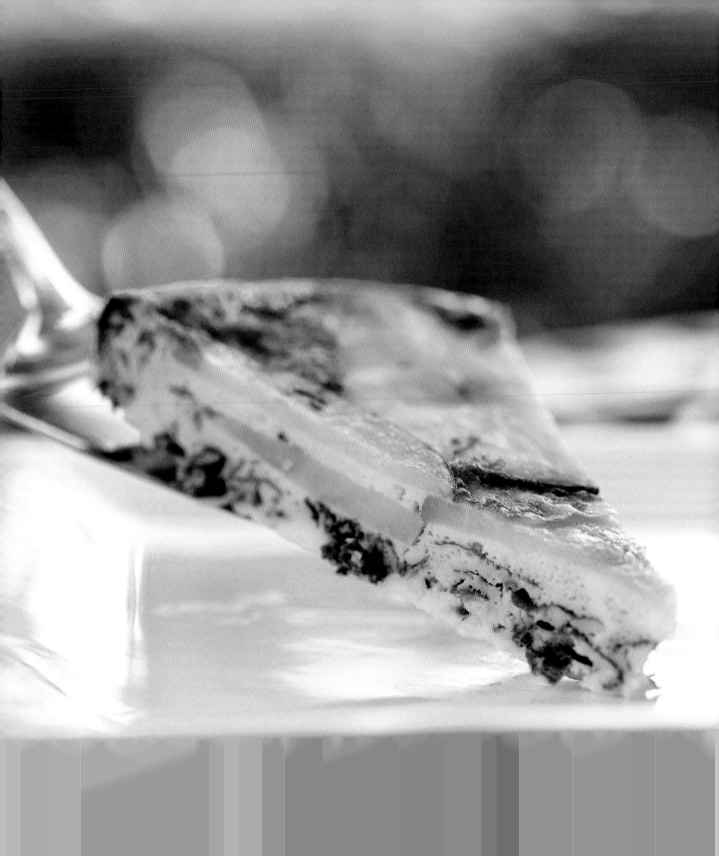

All-Star
KALE AND POTATO FRITTATA

FRITTATA WITH RED POTATOES, KALE AND PARMESAN

Who says kale isn't kid-friendly? When added to this absolutely yummy frittata, kale gets gobbled up! I know, firsthand. A frittata is a wonderful way to nourish the body and satisfy everyone's taste buds. When I describe a frittata, friends say, "Oh! It's an omelet," and while it may seem that way, there's a difference between the two. An omelet involves cooking the egg mixture first, then incorporating a filling, but when making a frittata, everything is mixed together in the sauté pan and the final product is usually served at room temperature. Technicalities aside, with healthy fats, savory ingredients and simple preparation, this recipe gets an A+ for nutrition and taste. Have leftovers? It makes a perfect and portable snack. Kids love to eat this cold, cut into bite-size pieces.

YIELD: 8 servings | **TIME:** 30 minutes

2 tbsp/30 ml extra-virgin olive oil

1 ½ cups/165 g red skinned new potatoes, sliced into ⅛"/3mm portions

Pinch of black pepper

¾ tsp salt, divided

5 cloves garlic, roughly chopped

1 cup/130 g cooked kale, chopped

½ tsp fresh thyme leaves, chopped

½ tsp fresh tarragon, chopped

8 eggs, beaten

1 oz/30 g Parmigiano-Reggiano, finely grated

Preheat oven to 350°F/180°C or gas mark 4. Heat olive oil over medium-high heat in a nonstick ovenproof 8-inch/20-centimeter sauté pan. Sauté potatoes, sprinkling with pepper and ¼ teaspoon of the salt, until browned, about 6 minutes. Add the garlic and cook for 30 seconds, or until aromatic. Stir in the kale to heat through. Stir the thyme, tarragon and remaining ½ teaspoon salt into the eggs. Pour them into the pan. Stir slowly with a wooden spoon or silicone spatula. As the egg starts to set, turn down the heat to low and stop stirring. Sprinkle with the Parmigiano-Reggiano. Transfer to oven and bake for about 10 minutes, or until the eggs are set and the cheese is lightly browned. Eggs are slightly jiggly when done. Allow to cool (the eggs will continue to cook and no longer jiggle) for 10 minutes. Slide the frittata onto a serving plate and cut into 6 or 8 wedges.

PER SERVING: Calories 140, protein 8 g, total fat 9 g, carbohydrates 7 g, sodium 350 mg, fiber 1 g

TINA'S TIP: Frittatas are a great way to use up leftovers or whatever is bountiful at the farmers' market. Just follow my basic method, and be creative! When I want to splurge on a heartier frittata, I omit the potatoes and use chicken sausage and onions instead.

Power Nutrient
PARFAIT

STONE FRUIT, PUMPKIN SEEDS, GREEK YOGURT AND GRANOLA PARFAIT

Stone fruits are one big healthy family, which includes cherries, plums, mangoes, apricots, nectarines and peaches. They get their name simply because their seeds resemble small stones. While they're always delicious eaten out of hand, I like to use them in parfaits. Or grill, roast or poach them. The antioxidants found in apricots actually become more available to the body when the fruit is cooked. Plums contribute vitamin K, which helps strengthen bones, and peaches offer potassium, a mineral that most people don't get enough of. In this parfait, the delicate sweetness of the fruit is enhanced that much more with some fresh rosemary, a glorious, aromatic herb that's also a source of important vitamins, minerals and phytonutrients. Nutrition aside, this parfait is eye candy, which makes it appealing to the entire family.

YIELD: 4 parfaits | **TIME:** 10 minutes

2 cups/475 g plain nonfat Greek yogurt

1 tsp/0.7 g fresh rosemary, finely chopped

¼ cup/60 ml honey

2 plums, peaches, or apricots or a combination of your favorite stone fruits, diced

2 cups/400 g granola

Stir the yogurt and rosemary together. Build the parfaits in glasses that hold at least 1 ¼ cups/320 milliliters. For each parfait, layer ¼ cup/60 g yogurt, 1 ½ teaspoons/7 milliliters honey, ¼ cup/40 grams fruit, ¼ cup/50 grams granola and repeat to create a second layer. Repeat for remaining glasses.

PER PARFAIT: Calories 300, protein 15 g, total fat 5 g, carbohydrates 51 g, sodium 65 mg, fiber 4 g

TINA'S TIP: This recipe is so versatile; it will work with nearly any fruit. Use what's in season, what you like and what looks best! If you prefer flavored yogurt, omit the honey.

Boost-My-Mood
BANANA SMOOTHIE

BLUEBERRY, BANANA AND YOGURT SMOOTHIE

Before a workout, this shake is nirvana for your body. The whey protein found in yogurt is an excellent source of amino acids, which provide energy for your muscles during exercise and, when combined with carbohydrates, produce the sustained energy you need to perform at your best. In addition, this shake contains 20 percent of your daily requirement for calcium, 25 percent of a day's worth of vitamin C, and two servings of phytochemical-rich fruit. If that isn't enough, the banana contributes potassium to help your body fend off muscle fatigue, and the almonds offer a nice dose of heart-healthy fats. Of course, it's delicious, too!

YIELD: 1 shake (about 10 oz/300 ml) | **TIME:** 5 minutes

¾ cup/109 g blueberries

½ banana

½ cup/120 g plain nonfat Greek yogurt

1 tbsp/16 g almond butter

2 tbsp/30 ml skim milk

Place all ingredients in a blender, and purée until smooth. Refrigerate blender container until shake is chilled, about 10 minutes. Purée on high and serve.

PER SERVING: Calories 250, protein 14 g, total fat 7 g, carbohydrates 38 g, sodium 110 mg, fiber 5 g

TINA'S TIP: Feel free to substitute almond milk for skim milk. It makes the shake lactose-free and enhances its overall flavor. Don't have blueberries on hand? Try blackberries or raspberries.

Make My **DATE**

DATE AND ALMOND MUFFINS

This recipe proves my theory that if you put anything in a muffin, a young child will eat it. Coming face to face with a date, my friend's toddler, Mia, wrinkled her nose and slowly backed away from the offending ingredient. Presented with the muffin, warm from the oven, Mia promptly ate two! Dates and orange zest give this mouthwatering muffin a delicious flavor, and the nuts provide a satisfying crunch—it's irresistible. While you might not be familiar with amaranth, a plant from which this nutritious, gluten-free flour is derived, you'll quickly come to love it. Amaranth flour is almost always mixed with other gluten-free flours to get successful results, and I like to incorporate it into my traditional muffin recipes to boost protein, calcium and iron content. Keep in mind that muffins aren't just for breakfast or brunch. I've even been known to pack them into brown bag lunches for dessert. Works every time!

YIELD: 12 muffins | **TIME:** 45 minutes

1 ¼ cups/150 g whole wheat flour

¾ cup/90 g amaranth flour

⅔ cup/150 g brown sugar, tightly packed

2 tsp/9 g baking powder

½ tsp baking soda

½ tsp salt

½ tsp cinnamon

1 tbsp/6 g orange zest

⅓ cup/80 ml orange juice

⅔ cup/160 ml buttermilk

1 egg

1 tsp/5 ml vanilla extract

4 tbsp/56 g unsalted butter, melted and cooled

⅔ cup/119 g sliced dates

1 cup/145 g toasted almonds, roughly chopped

Preheat oven to 375°F/190°C or gas mark 5. Line a 12-cup muffin pan with paper liners.

Place the whole wheat flour, amaranth flour, brown sugar, baking powder, baking soda, salt and cinnamon in a large bowl. Whisk together.

In another bowl, combine the orange zest, orange juice and buttermilk. Whisk in the egg, vanilla and butter. Whisk smooth. Add the dry ingredients in a couple of batches, stirring to combine with a rubber spatula or wooden spoon. Do not overmix or the muffins will become tough. Stir in the dates and almonds. Fill the muffin cups. Bake for 30 minutes, or until a toothpick inserted into the center comes out clean.

PER MUFFIN: Calories 240, protein 6 g, total fat 9 g, carbohydrates 35 g, sodium 250 mg, fiber 4 g

TINA'S TIP: For a change of pace, try baking this recipe in a loaf pan. Slice and serve as dessert with a scoop of vanilla frozen yogurt.

GREEN EGGS AND HAM
Torpedo

EGG, MOZZARELLA, SPINACH AND HAM BURRITO

More often than not, I feel like "Sam I Am," from the much-loved children's book, *Green Eggs and Ham*. Just like Sam, I spend considerable time trying to convince reluctant family members (whose names will not be mentioned here) to try something I've made, knowing full well, after a forkful is sampled, that the meal will be devoured. Inspired by Dr. Seuss, this breakfast, brunch or lunch burrito is packed with taste and nutrition. One serving delivers 45 percent of a day's worth of vitamin A, 20 percent of your daily need for iron, 25 percent of a day's worth of calcium and a good dose of high-quality protein. Oh, the wisdom of Dr. Seuss ...

YIELD: 4 servings | **TIME:** 20 minutes

6 oz/168 g spinach leaves

¼ cup/40 g chopped shallots

½ tsp thyme leaves

4 eggs

¼ tsp salt

Black pepper

2 (8"/20 cm) spinach tortillas

4 slices low-sodium ham

3 oz/84 g low-sodium fontina or mozzarella, grated

2 tsp/10 g unsalted butter

Microwave the spinach for 1 minute until wilted. Squeeze out excess liquid and roughly chop it. Place in a blender with the shallots, thyme and eggs. Season with salt and pepper to taste. Blend until the spinach is well incorporated, about 30 seconds.

Heat an 8-inch/20-centimeter nonstick pan over medium heat. Place 1 tortilla in the pan and allow it to brown on one side and puff slightly, about 30 seconds. Repeat on the second side. Reserve. Repeat with the second tortilla. Place 2 slices of ham on each tortilla and top with the cheese.

In the same pan, melt the butter, pour in the eggs and, using a silicone spatula or wooden spoon, push the eggs, allowing them to start to form large "curds" but not brown. Move them until they are set and not wet, 3 minutes. Divide the eggs between the tortillas, using the spatula to break up the eggs to mostly cover the tortilla, leaving a ½-inch/1.3-centimeter border. Roll up the tortilla and slice in half.

PER SERVING: Calories 270, protein 21 g, total fat 12 g, carbohydrates 21 g, sodium 500 mg, fiber 3 g

TINA'S TIP: Try using other greens such as broccoli in place of the spinach, or try adding a half bunch of cilantro to the mix and serve with salsa verde.

Lovin' **SPOONFUL**

BROILED GRAPEFRUIT WITH BROWN SUGAR AND AMARETTO

To borrow a phrase from my first book, I think this is the best breakfast recipe on the planet! While splashing your grapefruit with amaretto so early in the day may seem unusual, the alcohol from the liqueur burns off when cooked, and you're left with a sweet and simply sensational breakfast option. It's one I've enjoyed for decades, ever since my mother gave it to me when I was little. Serve the broiled grapefruit along with some oatmeal and milk, and you have a complete meal. Today, my family enjoys this very same dish, lapping up every bit of tasty grapefruit and skipping out the door. I'm just happy knowing they've gotten a good dose of vitamin C to enhance their immunity, antioxidants to prevent disease, pectin to keep blood sugar stable and a delicious meal that's evocative of their heritage.

YIELD: 4 servings | **TIME:** 10 minutes

2 ½ tbsp/35 g brown sugar

1 tbsp/15 ml amaretto liqueur

2 ruby red grapefruits

Preheat the broiler.

In a small bowl, add brown sugar, using your fingers to smooth out any lumps. Add amaretto, and using a spoon, combine until a paste forms. Then line a rimmed baking sheet with foil and set aside.

Using a serrated knife, cut each grapefruit lengthwise and then cut off the bottom of each grapefruit half so the grapefruit stays level. Turn the fruit upright, and using your knife, cut around the outside of the grapefruit flesh and make cuts to separate each segment. Then, place each grapefruit half on the foil-lined baking sheet. Layer sugar mixture evenly on each grapefruit. Place under the broiler. Broil until light brown on top, about 4 to 5 minutes. Remove from the oven. If any excess sugar mixture has dripped onto the baking sheet, spoon it over the grapefruit before serving.

PER SERVING: Calories 70, protein 1 g, total fat 0 g, carbohydrates 17 g, sodium 0 g, fiber 1 g

TINA'S TIP: Try using agave nectar, honey or raw sugar in place of the brown sugar for variation. Also, feel free to add a sprinkle of spice, such as ground ginger or cinnamon, for added flavor and nutrition.

Mother Nature's
GREEN MACHINE

JALAPEÑO-MINT SMOOTHIE

Even though it includes jalapeño, surprisingly, this smoothie really isn't hot at all—it's just loaded with flavor and healthy goodness. Green peppers, like jalapeño, contain an antioxidant called quercetin, which may decrease our body's ability to store fat. Combined with refreshing mint, creamy yogurt and a squeeze of agave nectar, this smoothie makes a great mid-morning snack. Greek yogurt contains fast-acting, extremely digestible whey protein that will help the body repair and build muscle, and in one serving you can enjoy 25 percent of a day's worth of calcium, 25 percent of your vitamin A needs and 20 percent of your vitamin C requirement.

YIELD: 2 servings | **TIME:** 10 minutes

1 ¼ tbsp/18 ml light agave nectar

½ tsp lime juice

3 tbsp/45 ml skim milk

2 cups/475 g plain nonfat Greek yogurt

1 jalapeño, seeded and sliced

⅓ cup/32 g fresh mint leaves, chopped, plus more for garnish (optional)

Pinch of salt

Combine all ingredients in a blender and blend until smooth. Don't be surprised if the mixture doesn't combine when you turn on the blender. Just stir it with a spoon to loosen it, then try and blend again. Repeat until the mixture is smoothie-smooth. Garnish with mint leaves, if desired. Serve immediately.

PER SERVING: Calories 190, protein 22 g, total fat 0 g, carbohydrates 25 g, sodium 230 mg, fiber 2 g

TINA'S TIP: Add the mint last so it's on top of the other ingredients, making it easier to blend. Otherwise, the mint has a tendency to tangle in the blender's blade.

Take-Me-Away
TROPICAL FRUIT SMOOTHIE

PINEAPPLE, COCONUT, BANANA AND MINT SMOOTHIE

After an especially challenging workout, I like to have a smoothie made with coconut milk; it's a rich source of magnesium, which helps alleviate soreness. Coconut milk is also known for its phosphorous content, and phosphorus works closely with calcium to strengthen bones and teeth. Just one serving of this crisp, refreshing and creamy smoothie will have you on the fast track to a stronger body!

YIELD: 1 serving (about 10 oz/300 ml)　　**TIME:** 5 minutes

5 oz/140 g pineapple, diced

½ banana, sliced

½ cup/120 ml low-fat coconut milk

2 tbsp/12 g chopped mint

1 tsp/5 ml lime juice

2 tbsp/30 ml ice water

Place all ingredients in a blender and purée until smooth. Chill the blender canister for 15 minutes in the freezer. Blend ingredients again, then serve immediately.

PER SERVING: Calories 216, protein 3 g, total fat 7 g, carbohydrates 39 g, sodium 23 mg, fiber 3 g

TINA'S TIP: If you're using fresh pineapple, cube the whole pineapple and freeze it on a baking tray. When frozen, place the cubes in a zip-top bag. You have fresh pineapple, at the ready, for whenever you may need it!

Best **PESTO SCRAMBLE**

EGG SCRAMBLE WITH BASIL PESTO

Everyone loves eggs. They're versatile, affordable, delicious and healthy. One whole egg has more nutrients per calorie than any other food, and eggs are a good source of quality protein, vitamin B12, selenium and riboflavin. Today, you can even buy eggs with more vitamin E, omega three fats and vitamin D. Science shows we can eat up to two eggs daily, without it affecting our cholesterol. Further, eggs are one of the best sources of choline, an element our body uses to break down fat, so eggs can really help you slim down or stay that way. This recipe harnesses the power of eggs and their satisfying taste by incorporating a bit of pesto and my "secret" ingredient, Greek yogurt! It will be a hit among young and old alike.

YIELD: 4 servings | **TIME:** 10 minutes

8 eggs

2 tbsp/30 g prepared pesto

½ cup/120 g low-fat Greek yogurt

Salt and pepper

2 tsp/10 ml extra-virgin olive oil

Whisk the eggs, pesto and yogurt together well. Season with salt and pepper to taste.

Heat a nonstick 8- to 10-inch/20- to 25-centimeter skillet over medium heat. Add the olive oil to coat the bottom and pour in the eggs. Use a rubber spatula and stir the eggs, allowing large curds to form. Continue to cook until the eggs are fully cooked or to desired consistency, about 8 minutes all together.

PER SERVING: Calories 220, protein 15 g, total fat 16 g, carbohydrates 3 g, sodium 150 mg, fiber 0 g

TINA'S TIP: If you'd like to serve this to adults, try substituting prepared olive tapenade for the pesto!

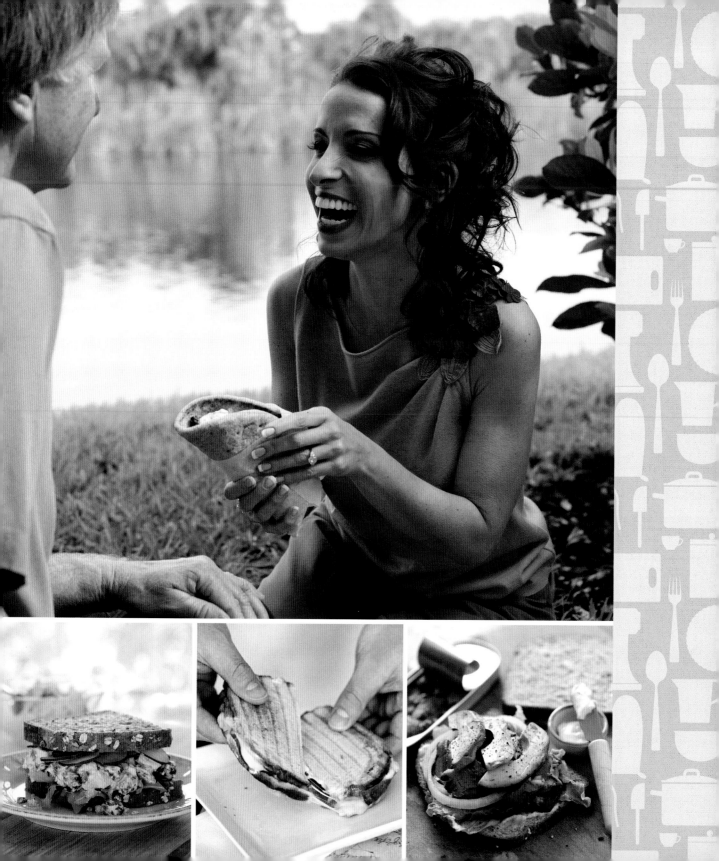

Easy-Peasy Panini and Sandwiches

Fill up, not out, with these scrumptious lunches!

Stacked, wrapped, grilled or pressed, sandwiches can't be beat! Hot or cold, they're satisfying, flavorful crowd-pleasers, and when you pair great bread with smart fillings, these recipes pack a wallop of vitamins, minerals and fiber.

Whether it's naan or panini, smørrbrød or muffaletta, these recipes are inspired by sandwiches from around the world. Some of my combinations know no restraint, where big, bold flavors spring from the bread; others are more demure. Some are for kids, others are not. Best of all, these sandwiches multitask for busy parents. Nearly all of the sandwiches can be enjoyed for a quick and easy dinner, and others can double as a snack when cut into pieces. No matter how you slice 'em (pun intended!), these sandwiches are packed with flavor and mega nutrition. This chapter is all about new, exciting, inspired ways to enjoy taste and health during that all-important midday meal.

Whether you're looking for the perfect picnic sandwich, something new for the old brown bag or a lunch that will make your child happy, these recipes will fill the bill. Set aside that ham and Swiss, step away from the peanut butter and jelly, and get ready to turn the ordinary into the extraordinary!

Two to **TANGO**

APPLE AND CHEDDAR QUESADILLA

Apples and cheese go together like peanut butter and jelly, but lovingly wrapped in a warm quesadilla and sprinkled with cumin, the fruit and cheese combination is taken beyond basic! And it's a real kid-pleaser because the cumin adds flavor that's over-the-top delicious without being overbearing. While making a few of these for the kids, make some for yourself by adding onions and chipotle purée. Packing 15 percent of a day's worth of calcium, antioxidants from the cumin—just ½ teaspoon has nearly two times as much as a carrot—and a generous serving of protein, this simple sandwich will instantly become a family go-to!

YIELD: 4 quesadillas | **TIME:** 15 minutes

1 tbsp/15 ml honey

1 tsp/5 ml chipotle purée (adult version)

¼ tsp ground cumin

1 cup/120 g grated Cheddar cheese

4 (8"/20 cm) flour tortillas

½ cup/80 g thinly sliced onion (adult version)

2 cups/220 g peeled and thinly sliced apple

Place honey, chipotle and cumin in a small bowl and stir to combine.

For each quesadilla, place a little less than ¼ cup/30 grams cheese on half the tortilla. Sprinkle with 2 tablespoons/20 grams onion, ½ cup/55 grams sliced apple, 1 teaspoon/5 milliliters reserved honey mixture and a little more cheese (this will act as "glue" to hold the ingredients together). Fold in half.

Heat a nonstick skillet over medium heat. Place quesadilla (heavy cheese side down) in the pan and cook for about 3 minutes, and then flip. Cook for 2 minutes more. Cheese should be melted and tortilla brown in spots and crisp. Cut into 4 wedges.

PER QUESADILLA: Calories 250, protein 12 g, total fat 5 g, carbohydrates 38 g, sodium 510 mg, fiber 4 g

TINA'S TIP: If you have a little extra time, it can be fun to infuse honey with herbs or spices, and it's a kid-friendly activity. Just place honey in a saucepan and add ground spices such as cumin or cinnamon, or try whole spices like clove or star anise. Then, warm the honey just until it starts to bubble, turn off heat and let sit for at least 15 minutes or longer. This step will "infuse" the honey with your chosen spice.

New Delhi **BELLY**

CURRIED POTATOES AND SPINACH IN NAAN

The flavors of Indian food are magical. They dance on your tongue, and the spice blends transform basic meat and vegetable dishes. Those spices also contribute to good health. Curcumin, a compound in curry, may have the power to lower breast cancer risk. Turmeric, another component of curry and nicknamed the "spice of life," may treat inflammatory diseases and protect our brain as we age. This Indian-inspired alternative to the standard sandwich will get you refueled in no time! Rich in protein and complex carbohydrates and packed with nearly a day's worth of vitamin A, this meal is complemented perfectly by a cooling cucumber-yogurt sauce. You could also serve this for supper, paired with a nice carrot-ginger or lentil soup.

YIELD: 4 servings | **TIME:** 30 minutes

½ lb/230 g potatoes, cut into ½"/1.3 cm chunks

2 tbsp/30 ml vegetable oil

1 cup/160 g finely chopped onion

1 tbsp/6.3 g curry powder

1 jalapeño, seeded and finely chopped

3 tbsp/24 g grated ginger

3 cloves garlic, finely chopped

1 lb/455 g spinach, stemmed and roughly chopped

Salt and pepper to taste

¾ cup/170 g plain Greek yogurt

½ cup/60 g grated hothouse cucumber

¼ tsp ground cumin

¼ cup/4 g cilantro, chopped

4 pieces naan bread, warmed according to package directions

Boil the potatoes in salted water until soft, about 7 minutes. Drain. Heat a large sauté pan over high heat. Add the oil and onion to the pan and lightly brown, about 5 minutes. Add the curry powder, jalapeño, ginger and garlic. Cook until aromatic, about 30 seconds. Add the spinach and cover the pan to wilt the spinach, about 3 minutes. Lower heat and stir in potatoes. Season with salt.

In a small bowl, combine the yogurt, cucumber, cumin and cilantro. Season with salt and pepper.

To assemble, place one-fourth of the spinach mixture in each naan. Drizzle with 3 tablespoons/45 milliliters of the yogurt sauce. Wrap the naan around the spinach and enjoy!

PER SERVING: Calories 280, protein 11 g, total fat 8 g, carbohydrates 41 g, sodium 310 mg, fiber 9 g

TINA'S TIP: Instead of spinach, try other vegetables such as mustard greens, finely sliced cauliflower or peas.

Extreme Makeover
CHICKEN SALAD SAMMY

CHICKEN, RED GRAPES, WALNUTS, DILL, SCALLIONS, RADISHES AND ARUGULA

When my mom comes to visit on a busy weekday, I want to make a quick yet nutritious lunch for the two of us. Chicken salad is a classic I can usually whip up using ingredients I have left over in my refrigerator. But this recipe is what I call a "basic made better." With less fat than traditional chicken salad, more protein and a lot more flavor, this luscious salad can be enjoyed on anything from a baguette to marbled rye or served in a pita or atop a bed of mixed greens with a side of cornbread. You can't go wrong! And it is all the better if you have cooked chicken on hand. Either way, you can make this satisfying lunch in a snap.

YIELD: 4 sandwiches | **TIME:** 25 minutes

8 oz/224 g chicken breast

½ cup/75 g red grapes, quartered

2 tbsp/14 g toasted walnuts, roughly chopped

2 tbsp/8 g dill, roughly chopped

¼ cup/25 g finely chopped scallion

½ cup/120 g low-fat Greek yogurt

¼ tsp salt

Several grates of freshly ground black pepper

8 slices multigrain bread

2 cups/40 g arugula

1 cup/116 g thinly sliced radishes

To cook the chicken, bring a saucepan of water to a boil over high heat. Add the chicken and simmer for 15 minutes, or until cooked through. Remove from water and cool completely. When cool, cut into ½-inch/1.3-centimeter dice. Place in a bowl with the grapes, walnuts, dill, scallions, yogurt, salt and black pepper. Stir to combine.

To assemble the sandwiches, place 4 slices of bread on a work surface. For each sandwich, top with ½ cup/10 grams arugula, ½ cup/70 grams chicken salad, ¼ cup/29 grams sliced radishes and another piece of bread.

You can also try substituting shrimp for the chicken and hazelnuts for the walnuts!

PER SANDWICH: Calories 260, protein 23 g, total fat 6 g, carbohydrates 28 g, sodium 460 mg, fiber 5 g

TINA'S TIP: Save the cooking water from the chicken. It will be lightly flavored from the chicken and can make a nice base broth for soup. Freeze it!

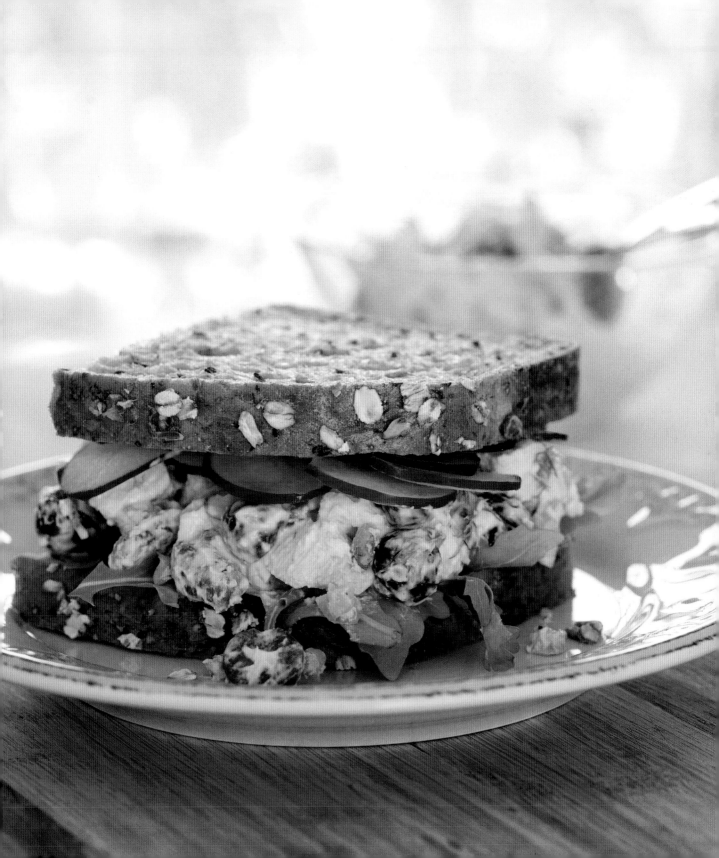

SQUEEZE Me!

PRESSED SANDWICH WITH ROASTED TOMATOES

In Italy, as in so many other European nations, a child's lunch is considered to be an integral part of their education. They learn about their regional cuisine, they cultivate tastes for a broad array of foods, and they make the most of the midday meal to nourish their young, growing bodies. The last time I was in Italy, I visited a school during pranzo, or lunch, and the children were gobbling up pasta, fish, veggies and fruit. Eating a sandwich for lunch in Italy is not as popular as it is Stateside, but there's no doubt American children love Italian food. So, I blended the best of both worlds—the flavors of Italy with the convenience of the American sandwich—and came up with this mouthwatering pressed sandwich that's a hit in my home. I promise it will become a favorite in yours, too!

YIELD: 4 servings | **TIME:** 45 minutes

---

3 plum tomatoes

2 tsp/10 ml olive oil, divided

Salt and pepper

¼ tsp thyme leaves

2 tsp/6 g finely chopped garlic

8 medium asparagus spears

8 slices sourdough bread

4 oz/112 g fresh mozzarella, thinly sliced (preferably no salt added)

4 tsp/20 ml basil pesto

Preheat oven to 400°F/200°C or gas mark 6. Trim the stem ends from the tomatoes, then slice crosswise into a total of 12 slices. Brush a baking tray with a small amount of olive oil. Place the tomato slices on the tray and sprinkle with a little bit of salt and pepper. Turn them over and repeat. Sprinkle with the thyme and garlic. Place in the oven and roast until tomatoes and garlic have started to brown slightly and much of their water content has evaporated, about 30 minutes. Remove from oven and set aside.

Roast the asparagus at the same time. Trim the tough white or purple stems from the asparagus and discard. Measure the asparagus to fit the length of the bread. Save extra pieces to make soup. Place the asparagus on a lightly oiled baking tray. Sprinkle with a little salt and pepper. Roast for about 10 minutes, or until softened and bright green, about 10 minutes. When cool enough to handle, slice in half lengthwise. Set aside.

To assemble the sandwiches, place 4 slices of bread on a work surface. For each sandwich, top with 1 ounce/28 grams mozzarella, 3 slices tomato and 4 pieces asparagus. Spread 1 teaspoon/5 milliliters pesto on remaining slices bread. Close sandwiches and brush both sides with a small amount of olive oil. Place in a panini press and cook until golden and cheese is melted, about 4 minutes.

PER SANDWICH: Calories 330, protein 17 g, total fat 10 g, carbohydrates 44 g, sodium 490 mg, fiber 4 g

TINA'S TIP: The tomatoes in this recipe are so delicious you'll want to have them on hand for other dishes. They're great on a burger or in a salad. Additionally, roasting hothouse tomatoes makes them taste more flavorful.

Rising Sun **PORK BUN**

CHAR SUI PORK SANDWICH

I love bao, and if you've never tried one, you must. Bao is Cantonese and means "bun," and it's essentially a soft, steamed roll filled with sweet, succulent, barbecued pork tenderloin. You can find bao on the menu of good Chinese restaurants, and it's usually served as dim sum. Inspired by traditional bao, this recipe is loaded with flavor and fun to eat. Recently, I served this sandwich to a pack of hungry teenage boys, and every morsel was devoured! Nutritious and tasty, pork is a high-protein, low-fat meat that helps maintain lean body mass. While this pork sandwich makes a delicious lunch, it can also double as a satisfying dinner when paired with a green salad or coleslaw.

YIELD: 6 sandwiches | **TIME:** 35 minutes

12 oz/340 g pork tenderloin

Salt and pepper

½ tsp five-spice powder

1 cup/100 g finely chopped scallion

6 tbsp/90 ml hoisin sauce

2 tbsp/30 ml low-sodium soy sauce

1 tbsp/15 ml honey

1 tbsp/8 g grated ginger

1 tbsp/10 g grated garlic

6 tbsp/90 ml plus 2 tsp/10 ml rice vinegar, divided

2 cups/140 g coleslaw mix

6 (6"/15 cm) whole wheat hero rolls

Preheat oven to 400°F/200°C or gas mark 6. Sprinkle tenderloin with salt and pepper. Place on a baking sheet and cook until an instant-read thermometer reaches 155°F/68°C, about 15 minutes. Let rest for 5 minutes before slicing crosswise first into ¼-inch/6-millimeter slices, then each slice into ¼-inch/6-millimeter strips.

While pork is cooking, place five-spice powder, scallion, hoisin, soy sauce, honey, ginger, garlic and 6 tablespoons/90 milliliters of the rice vinegar into a small saucepan. Stir to combine and simmer for 5 minutes, or until thickened slightly. Toss the sauce with the reserved pork.

In another bowl, toss the coleslaw mix with the remaining 2 teaspoons/10 milliliters rice vinegar and a sprinkle of salt or soy sauce. Set aside.

Slice the rolls in half and toast if desired. Place on a work surface. Divide the coleslaw mix among the bottom half of the rolls, then top with the pork. Close the sandwiches and serve.

PER SERVING: Calories 290, protein 19 g, total fat 6 g, carbohydrates 43 g, sodium 560 mg, fiber 6 g

TINA'S TIP: Try serving the pork mixture in Boston lettuce cups as an hors d'oeuvre or snack.

The Scandalous
SCANDINAVIAN

SMOKED SALMON, HARD-BOILED EGG, TOMATOES, GREENS AND CAPER-ONION MAYO

This is another one of those fabulous "adult sandwiches" that I mention on page 45. It's hearty enough to pack for work, yet it's perfectly appropriate for a luncheon or brunch. The hardest part of this recipe is assembling the ingredients: that's how easy it is, yet it tastes like a gourmet sandwich you'd find on a restaurant menu or at a specialty deli. Thanks to the salmon, the sandwich is loaded with omega-3 fatty acids that our body can't make on its own; it's high in protein and delivers a whopping amount of nutrients per calorie. In other words, it's the heavyweight nutrition champ of sandwiches!

YIELD: 4 sandwiches | **TIME:** 25 minutes

2 large eggs

1 tbsp/14 g low-fat mayonnaise

1 tbsp/14 g low-fat Greek yogurt

2 tsp/8 g grainy mustard

1 tbsp/8.6 g finely chopped capers

1 tbsp/4 g dill, roughly chopped, plus more for garnish

2 tbsp/20 g finely chopped red onion

Several grates of freshly ground black pepper

4 pieces pumpernickel bread

2 cups/40 g mixed greens

8 thin slices beefsteak tomato

8 oz/230 g smoked salmon

To make hard-boiled eggs, place the eggs in a saucepan and cover with water. Bring to a boil, then turn off the heat and let sit for 12 minutes. Rinse in cool water. When cool enough to handle, peel the eggs and rinse off any bits of shell. Cut each egg into 8 wedges. Set aside.

To make the caper-onion mayonnaise, combine the mayonnaise, yogurt, grainy mustard, capers, dill, red onion and black pepper in a bowl. Set aside.

To assemble the sandwiches, toast the bread, if desired, and place on a work surface. For each sandwich, spread 2 teaspoons/8 grams caper-onion mayonnaise on each slice bread. Top with ½ cup/10 grams greens, 2 slices tomato, 2 ounces/56 grams smoked salmon and 4 wedges of egg. Sprinkle with additional dill.

PER SANDWICH: Calories 340, protein 41 g, total fat 11 g, carbohydrates 19 g, sodium 440 mg, fiber 3 g

TINA'S TIP: The caper-onion mayonnaise makes more than you'll use in this recipe, so save it! It's delicious in tuna fish. Try it in your next tuna salad.

Get Your **JAM ON**

GRILLED CHEESE WITH STRAWBERRY JAM

If there's a recipe that will make you melt, this is it! Soft, warm cheese is the perfect complement to crusty multigrain bread, and a dollop of jam adds a burst of sweetness to the savory flavor of the Cheddar. Not only is this sandwich delicious, but it also offers a good dose of protein and fiber and 35 percent of a day's worth of bone-building calcium. Authentic farmhouse Cheddar is a yellow-beige color, but don't be afraid of the American-made orange variety. It's colored with annatto, which is a spice used to give Cheddar its signature color.

YIELD: 4 sandwiches | **TIME:** 15 minutes

8 slices multigrain bread

4 tbsp/80 g low-sugar strawberry jam

4 oz/115 g Cheddar cheese, sliced

Unsalted butter, for cooking

To assemble the sandwiches, place 4 slices of bread on a work surface. Spread 1 tablespoon/20 grams strawberry jam on 4 slices of bread. Top with 1 ounce/28 grams of the Cheddar and top with another slice of bread. Close sandwiches and brush both sides with a small amount of butter. Heat a large nonstick pan over medium heat. Place the sandwiches in the pan and cook until golden, about 3 minutes. Press on the sandwiches to help "glue" them together. Turn them and cook on the second side until golden, another 3 minutes.

PER SANDWICH: Calories 190, protein 12 g, total fat 5 g, carbohydrates 36 g, sodium 610 mg, fiber 10 g

TINA'S TIP: You don't need much butter to crisp and brown the outside of these sandwiches. Melt the butter before you brush the bread with it and it will be much easier to evenly coat without saturating the bread.

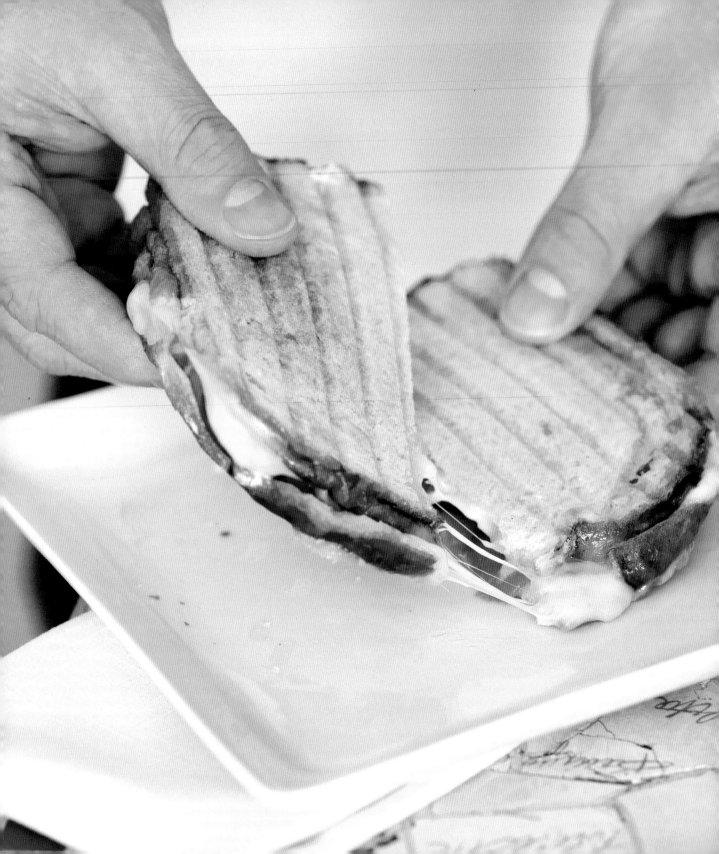

Parma **PANINI**

PRESSED SANDWICH WITH HAM, PEACHES, ROASTED RED PEPPER AND GRUYÈRE

This is my go-to sandwich when I have only five minutes to make a meal. When time is tight, most people snack, but why nosh on empty calories when you can eat something that will add significant nutrients to your daily diet? This grown-up sandwich offers 25 percent of a day's worth of vitamin A, 40 percent of a day's worth of calcium and 60 percent of your requirement for vitamin C. It's chock-full of protein, fiber and nearly thirty different types of carotenoids from the red pepper. Bon appetit!

YIELD: 4 sandwiches | **TIME:** 15 minutes

8 slices multigrain bread

4 oz/115 g Gruyère, thinly sliced

4 oz/115 g smoked ham, thinly sliced

4 oz/115 g roasted red pepper, roughly chopped

1 medium peach, pitted and thinly sliced

4 tsp/20 g grainy mustard

Unsalted butter, melted, for brushing on bread

To assemble the sandwiches, place 4 slices of bread on a work surface. Top each slice with 1 or 2 slices of Gruyère, 2 slices of ham, 1 ounce/28 grams roasted red pepper and 2 slices of peach. Spread 1 teaspoon/5 grams grainy mustard on each of the remaining slices of bread and close the sandwiches. Using a pastry brush, brush a small amount of butter on both sides of the sandwiches. Place in a sandwich press or panini maker and cook until golden on the outside and warm with melted cheese on the inside.

If you want to make your own roasted red peppers, it's easy. Simply place the pepper directly on the open flame of the stove. Using tongs, turn the pepper so that it's blistered and blackened on all sides. Remarkably, this won't set off the smoke alarm! Place in a bowl and cover with plastic wrap until cool enough to handle. The skins will slip right off. Slice in half to remove the seeds. Rinse. Keep refrigerated until ready to use.

PER SANDWICH: Calories 290, protein 19 g, total fat 12 g, carbohydrates 35 g, sodium 720 mg, fiber 11 g

TINA'S TIP: If fresh peaches aren't available, try substituting a spoonful of prepared mango chutney!

Caribbean **SAMMY**

CUMIN SHRIMP, AVOCADO, MASHED BLACK BEANS, ORANGES AND GREENS

Fresh sandwich ideas are always welcome in my home. Standard options get tired quickly, and growing teens with hardy appetites demand sustenance, novelty and lots of nutrition. This recipe fires on all cylinders, packing filling ingredients, an inspired combination of textures and flavors and mega nutrition into each bite! The shrimp and beans offer protein and fiber, the oranges add a punch of vitamin C and the avocado contributes heart-healthy vitamin E and glutathione, a powerful antioxidant that is suspected of fighting disease. Of course, it tastes delicious!

YIELD: 4 servings | **TIME:** 25 minutes

---

16 medium shrimp, peeled and deveined

1 tsp/5 ml vegetable oil

2 tsp/8 g grated garlic, divided

¾ tsp ground cumin, divided

¼ tsp salt, plus extra for sprinkling

1 (15 oz/420 g) can black beans, drained and rinsed

¼ cup/40 g finely diced red onion

2 tbsp/30 ml water

2 tbsp/30 ml lime juice, divided

1 orange, peeled and pulled into segments and roughly chopped

4 (6"/15 cm) pieces baguette

4 leaves romaine lettuce

½ avocado, thinly sliced

3 tbsp/3 g cilantro, roughly chopped

Place the shrimp in a bowl with the oil, 1 teaspoon/4 grams of the garlic, ¼ teaspoon of the cumin and a sprinkle of salt. Reserve.

To make the beans, place them in a saucepan with the red onion, remaining 1 teaspoon/4 grams garlic, remaining ½ teaspoon cumin, the ¼ teaspoon salt, the water and 1 tablespoon/15 milliliters of the lime juice. Heat over low heat and use a whisk or fork to mash the beans and mix ingredients. Be sure to leave some beans whole. Remove from heat and reserve.

Heat a pan over low to medium heat. Add the shrimp and cook, stirring until they are pink and cooked through, about 3 minutes. Stir in the remaining 1 tablespoon/15 milliliters lime juice and chopped orange segments. Season with a sprinkle of salt if needed. Reserve.

To assemble the sandwiches, slice the baguettes in half lengthwise and toast if desired. Place the bottoms on a work surface. Spread one-fourth of the bean mixture along the bottom of the baguettes. Top with 1 lettuce leaf, a few slices avocado, one-fourth of the shrimp and orange mixture and a sprinkle of cilantro. Top with the other half of the baguette.

PER SANDWICH: Calories 280, protein 21 g, total fat 6 g, carbohydrates 37 g, sodium 300 mg, fiber 9 g

TINA'S TIP: This sandwich will also work well in a whole wheat hoagie or other hardy bread.

TUNA Tune-Up

OIL-PACKED TUNA, HARD-BOILED EGG, ROASTED FENNEL, TOMATOES, TAPENADE AND GREENS

Lots of cookbooks offer creative ideas for kids' lunches, but what about the rest of us? Lunch can get tiresome for adults, too, so I decided to create a few sandwich recipes for an older crowd—ideas that will get you out of your same-old-sandwich rut, amp up your midday nutrition, and energize you for the demands of the afternoon. If you want a change of pace, this recipe is for you! It's basically egg salad dressed up for an evening out, and it's absolutely delicious! It's loaded with omega-3 fatty acids that keep the brain sharp and help performance, plus protein from the tuna and egg and antioxidants from the fennel; the flavor is over the top! Cook the fennel over the weekend, so you have it on hand to enjoy during the week.

YIELD: 4 sandwiches | **TIME:** 40 minutes, including cooking time

1 bulb fennel

1 tsp/5 ml olive oil

Salt and pepper

2 large eggs

4 (4"/10 cm) pieces of baguette, sliced in half

4 tsp/20 g tapenade

2 cups/40 g mesclun

4 thick slices beefsteak tomato

6 oz/168 g olive oil-packed tuna, drained

Preheat oven to 400°F/200°C or gas mark 6. Remove dark green stalks from the fennel and reserve for another use (see tip). Cut the fennel in half lengthwise, then into ⅓-inch/8-millimeter slices crosswise. Place on a baking sheet and toss with the olive oil and a little salt and pepper. Roast until softened and lightly browned in some areas, about 30 minutes.

To make hard-boiled eggs, place the eggs in a saucepan and cover with water. Bring to a boil, and then turn off the heat and let sit for 12 minutes. Rinse in cool water. When cool enough to handle, peel the eggs and rinse off any bits of shell. Cut each egg into 8 wedges. Reserve.

To assemble the sandwiches, place the bottom of the baguettes on a work surface. Spread each with 1 teaspoon/5 grams tapenade. Top with ½ cup/10 grams mesclun, 1 slice tomato, 1 ½ ounces/42 grams fennel, 1 ½ ounces/42 grams tuna and 4 wedges of egg. Top with other half of baguette.

PER SANDWICH: Calories 210, protein 19 g, total fat 8 g, carbohydrates 15 g, sodium 350 mg, fiber 3 g

TINA'S TIP: Don't throw out those fennel stalks! The fennel stalks have great flavor, but they can be a little tough. What to do with them? Make vegetable stock! Simmer them in water with any other vegetables scraps like onion tops and skin, carrot peels, and stems from herbs. (Yup. Stuff you'd put in the composter.) Vegetable stock doesn't take more than 30 minutes of simmering and adds fabulous depth of flavor to soups, sauces and risotto, and it freezes beautifully.

Tasty **TRIO**

NUTELLA, GRANOLA AND FRUIT QUESADILLA

My childhood friend was of German heritage, and I vividly recall—in the third grade—her opening up her little metal lunchbox to reveal the chocolate sandwich her mother had made. I thought that was the coolest thing. I was eager to try a bite, and when I did, I was hooked. It's one of those food memories I've never forgotten. Inspired by that memory, I created a modern-day chocolate sandwich that's as fun to make as it is to eat. Brimming with colorful fresh fruit, it's an effective way to get a child to eat a serving of fruit. The chocolate spread complements the fruit, adding a wonderful texture and aroma, and a little sprinkling of granola gives this quesadilla an unexpected but yummy crunch!

YIELD: 2 servings | **TIME:** 10 minutes

2 (8"/20 cm) whole wheat tortillas

2 tbsp/32 g chocolate-hazelnut spread

1 cup/150 g finely chopped mixed fruit (such as bananas, pears and strawberries)

2 tbsp/28 g granola

Heat a nonstick skillet over medium heat. Place 1 tortilla in the pan and spread 1 tablespoon/16 grams chocolate-hazelnut spread over half of it. Sprinkle with half the fruit and 1 tablespoon/14 grams of the granola. Fold the tortilla in half and continue to cook until crisp and golden in spots, about 2 minutes. Flip tortilla and crisp the second side, about 1 minute. Repeat with other tortilla. Cut each tortilla into 4 triangles.

PER QUESADILLA: Calories 210, protein 3 g, total fat 7 g, carbohydrates 35 g, sodium 55 mg, fiber 3 g

TINA'S TIP: Other additions that would be nice include toasted coconut or nuts. In place of the chocolate-hazelnut spread, you can try a nut butter (almond or peanut) and dark chocolate chips.

Happy **VEGGIE POCKET**

HOMEMADE HUMMUS PITA

My family loves hummus, but it's loaded with oil, and the commercial varieties are expensive compared with the cost of making it yourself. Plus, preparing it at home is a great way to introduce young children to cooking; there's no chopping involved and everything gets whirled in a food processor. Easy! Just one bite of my healthy hummus, which incorporates flaxseeds and replaces oil with Greek yogurt, and you will be hooked on making hummus at home. Of course, it goes without saying this meal is chock-full of nutrients your body needs to stay healthy. Sprouts are important for cellular regeneration; flaxseeds are a vegan source of essential omega-3 fatty acids; tahini offers B vitamins and cancer-fighting calcium; and chickpeas provide fiber. Eat up!

YIELD: 6 servings, 3½ cups/788 g hummus | **TIME:** 20 minutes

2 (15½ oz/434 g) cans chickpeas, rinsed and drained

2½ tbsp/37.5 ml lemon juice

1 tbsp/15 g tahini

½ tsp kosher salt

½ cup/112 g nonfat Greek yogurt

2 tbsp/30 g ground flaxseed

5 tbsp/75 ml water

6 pita halves

1 cup/50 g alfalfa sprouts

1 cup/110 g grated carrot

1 medium cucumber, peeled and diced

In a food processor, add chickpeas, lemon juice, tahini, salt, yogurt and flaxseed. Begin to purée mixture, pouring water through the feeder tube of processor as it processes until mixture becomes smooth. If needed, add 1 or 2 tablespoons/15 or 30 milliliters of additional water to get the hummus to desired consistency. Taste the hummus, adding more salt or lemon juice to season if needed. Stuff pitas with hummus, alfalfa sprouts, carrots and cucumbers, and serve. Use remaining hummus as a dip for vegetables.

PER 1 TABLESPOON/14 GRAMS HUMMUS: Calories 15, protein 1 g, total fat 0 g, carbohydrates 2 g, sodium 35 mg, fiber 1 g

PER ONE PITA HALF WITH VEGGIES AND ¼ CUP/56 GRAMS HUMMUS: Calories 150, protein 5 g, total fat 1 g, carbohydrates 20 g, sodium 195 mg, fiber 5 g

TINA'S TIP: For adult consumption, I like to add hot sauce to my hummus. The fiery flavor will wake up your taste buds and add a depth of flavor to this rich and satisfying spread.

KIPPERS and Bits

KIPPERS, VIDALIA ONIONS, LEMONY MAYO AND GREENS

When I went to Norway two years ago, I was amazed by how healthy everyone looked. The women, in particular, had complexions that were milky white; their hair was shiny, and they had a radiance about them that could only come from the incredible amounts of omega-3-rich, cold-water fish they ate. When I returned home, I tried to maintain a high level of fish consumption, knowing it would also be beneficial for my brain, heart and muscle mass. Scientifically speaking, the protective effects of fish consumption greatly outweigh any of the risks you may read about. This recipe was inspired by my trip to Norway, and it's as delicious as it is nutritious; the sandwich is bursting with heart-healthy fats, vitamins D and A and the minerals calcium and potassium. Kippers are salted, cold-smoked herring; if you can't find them, try sardines or anchovies. While this meal isn't the most kid-friendly, it will keep you nourished and energized so you can tackle whatever life throws your way!

YIELD: 4 sandwiches | **TIME:** 20 minutes

2 tbsp/30 g low-fat mayonnaise

1 tbsp/15 ml nonfat Greek yogurt

⅛ tsp lemon zest

1 tsp/5 ml lemon juice

4 slices multigrain bread

4 leaves crisp lettuce (such as Boston, romaine or Bibb)

4 thick slices beefsteak tomato

4 thin slices Vidalia onion

2 (3 ¼ oz/91 g) cans kippers, drained

4 oz/112 g avocado, thinly sliced (optional)

Freshly ground black pepper, to taste

Combine the mayonnaise, yogurt, lemon zest and juice. Set aside.

Toast the bread. To assemble the sandwiches, place the bread on a work surface and spread with the lemony sauce. Top with 1 leaf of lettuce (fold it if necessary), 1 slice of tomato, 1 slice of onion, one-fourth of the kipper filets and 1 ounce/28 grams of the avocado. Season with freshly ground black pepper.

PER SANDWICH: Calories 380, protein 17 g, total fat 19 g, carbohydrates 37 g, sodium 690 mg, fiber 12 g

TINA'S TIP: Kippers on toast is a classic meal in Great Britain and Ireland, while sardines are more popular in Scandinavia. Either fish works in this recipe, and if you have leftovers, toss them into eggs, a salad or a red sauce for a punch of flavor!

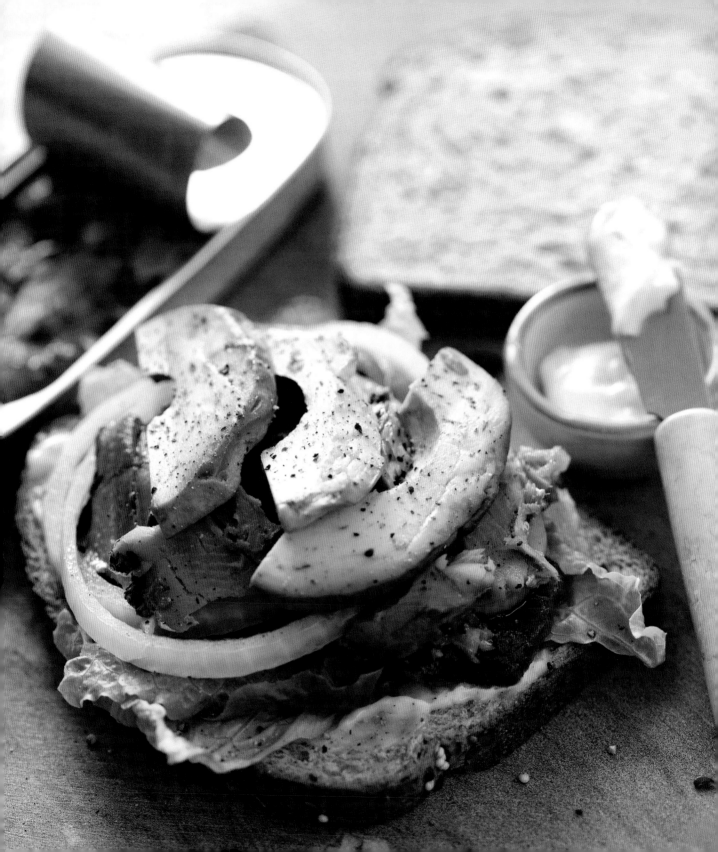

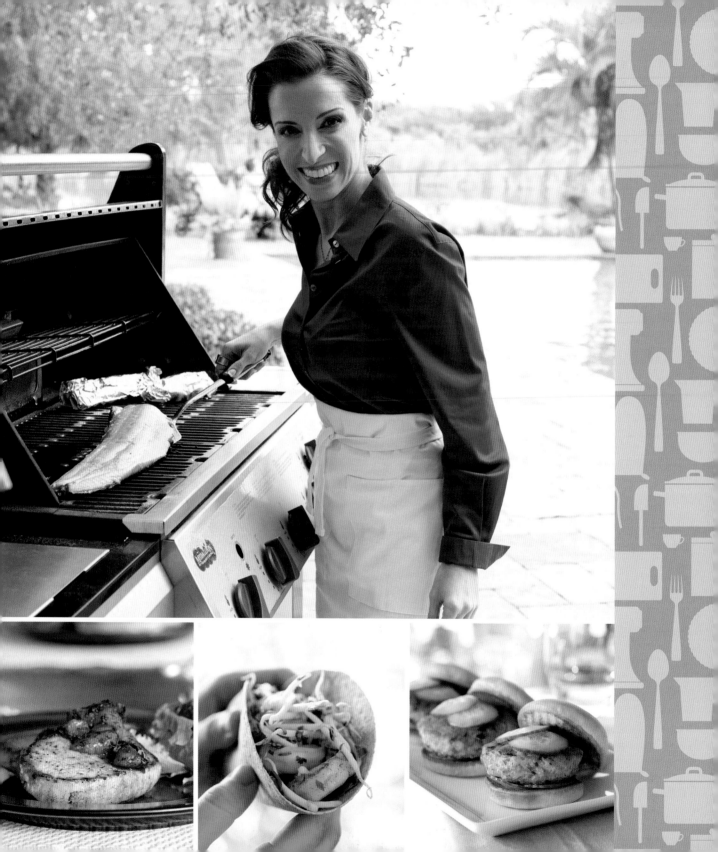

Power Proteins from Land and Sea

More flavor, fewer calories, better health. Bring it!

Today, going meatless, raw or macrobiotic is trendy, but so is eating a very high-protein diet. On the Web, in books and on television, experts passionately argue their nutrition ideologies and subsequently, people adopt polar beliefs. Among nutritionists, there seems to be no other topic that inspires so much debate.

My nutrition philosophy is a hybrid of the two lifestyles; I don't plan to give up eating meat, but you surely won't find me serving my family excessive amounts of protein and eliminating grains and legumes in the process.

There are elements of vegan diets that I like, and there are aspects of the popular Paleo diet that have relevance, so the recipes in this chapter find harmony between the two divergent approaches to wellness.

If you come to my house for dinner, you'll see my philosophy in practice. For example, my Simply Savory Stuffed Pork is a creative way to use a small amount of meat, and it reflects my grand-mother's culinary influence, as well as her intent to nourish her family in the best way possible. In essence, small portions of meat, poultry or fish combined with the freshest ingredients possible deliver superlative flavors and mega nutrition to the friends and family around my table.

So, pick up your knife and fork! Dig into my mouthwatering baked spaghetti squash with chicken sausage, mini salmon sliders and pork tenderloin with peach chutney, and taste how proteins and produce can coexist in peace.

FULL 'n' PLENTY

STUFFED CHICKEN WITH HERBED RICOTTA AND KALE

Chicken is a natural choice when I want to make a quick and healthy meal for my family. A single serving of poultry provides half of a day's worth of high-quality protein, and it's a good source of vitamins and minerals, including phosphorous and zinc. Chicken never gets boring, because it's available in a variety of cuts, and you can dress it up or down. The results of this recipe are impressive. It'll receive "oohs" and "ahhs" at the table; you'll feel like a professional chef! Using just a few, fresh ingredients, you can turn simple into sensational with little effort and less time. The chicken is tender, juicy and nutritious, delivering 45 percent of your vitamin A needs, 30 percent of a day's worth of vitamin C and 20 percent of your iron requirement. Now that's pretty close to perfect.

YIELD: 4 servings | **TIME:** 35 minutes

¼ cup/17 g roughly chopped Tuscan kale (about 3 leaves)

½ cup/120 g part-skim ricotta

2 tsp/6 g grated garlic

½ tsp fresh rosemary leaves, finely chopped

½ tsp fresh oregano leaves, finely chopped

¼ cup/25 g grated Parmigiano-Reggiano

½ tsp salt, plus additional for seasoning

2 (8 oz/224 g) boneless, skinless chicken breasts

Freshly ground pepper

2 tsp/10 ml vegetable oil

Place a small saucepan of salted water over high heat and bring to a boil. Add the Tuscan kale and simmer until tender, about 5 minutes, depending on how mature the kale is. Drain the kale. When cool enough to handle, finely chop the kale. Transfer to a bowl along with the ricotta, garlic, rosemary, oregano, Parmigiano-Reggiano and the ½ teaspoon salt. Mix well. Reserve.

Butterfly the chicken. Place chicken breast on a cutting board. Using a sharp knife, preferably a chef's knife or a boning knife, hold it parallel to the cutting surface, and carefully cut the breast in half, leaving a "hinge" the length of the breast. Repeat with other breast. Place half of the ricotta filling on one side of each breast. Close the breast and use toothpicks (3 per breast should do it) to "sew" the breast closed, or you can use a bamboo skewer.

Preheat oven to 400°F/200°C or gas mark 6. Heat an ovenproof sauté pan over medium-high heat. Season the chicken on both sides with a little salt and pepper. Add the oil to the pan, and then brown the chicken for about 2 minutes on each side. Transfer to the oven and cook 10 minutes (an instant-read thermometer should read 165°F/73°C). Let rest 5 minutes before removing the toothpicks. Cut each breast on the diagonal into 8 slices and serve 4 slices per person.

PER SERVING: Calories 270, protein 34 g, total fat 14 g, carbohydrates 4 g, sodium 390 mg, fiber 0 g

TINA'S TIP: These are elegant enough for a dinner party but also make a delicious weeknight dinner. The bonus is that they can be assembled ahead of time and frozen, so make extra to have on hand.

Peachy PORK

TENDERLOIN WITH PEACH CHUTNEY

For most people, eating healthier usually means eliminating something from their diet, such as fat or sugar, but that doesn't have to be the case. A "healthy" meal need not consist of plain, grilled chicken. Who wants to eat that? Not me. To eat nutritiously, I usually add something to a dish so it provides more vitamins, minerals and essential nutrients. In this recipe, I add chutney! This savory and hearty chutney pumps up the flavor and the overall nutrient profile of the meal, and it adds a natural sweetness that kids love. Since the chutney lasts awhile in the refrigerator, I usually double the recipe and have it on hand for nights I make poultry or pork.

YIELD: 6 servings (chutney yields 1 ½ cups/375 g)　|　**TIME:** 40 minutes

1 lb/455 g peaches, diced

¼ cup/36 g raisins

¼ cup/60 ml cider or sherry vinegar

½ cup/115 g dark brown sugar, packed

½ cup/80 g finely chopped onion

2 tsp/6 g finely chopped garlic

2 tsp/5 g grated ginger

½ tsp salt, divided

6 (4 oz/112 g) pieces pork tenderloin

Freshly ground pepper

3 tbsp/21 g ground cumin

1 tbsp/15 ml vegetable oil

Place the peaches, raisins, vinegar, brown sugar, onion, garlic, ginger and ¼ teaspoon salt in a nonreactive saucepan. Bring to a simmer and cook over low heat for about 30 minutes, or until the juices have thickened into a syrup.

Preheat oven to 400°F/200°C or gas mark 6. While the chutney is cooking, prepare the pork. Sprinkle the pork with the remaining ¼ teaspoon salt, pepper to taste, and cumin. Roll the pork in the cumin, pressing it so it's completely covered.

Heat an ovenproof sauté pan over medium heat. Add the vegetable oil and lightly brown the pork on all sides, about 5 minutes. Transfer the pan to the oven. Cook for 10 minutes for medium. Serve with ¼ cup/65 g chutney.

PER SERVING: Calories 250, protein 17 g, total fat 5 g, carbohydrates 34 g, sodium 390 mg, fiber 3 g

TINA'S TIP: Chutney keeps for 3 months in the refrigerator, and it's a great way to use any type of stone fruit you may have on hand. Give it a try with plums, nectarines, apricots or mangos!

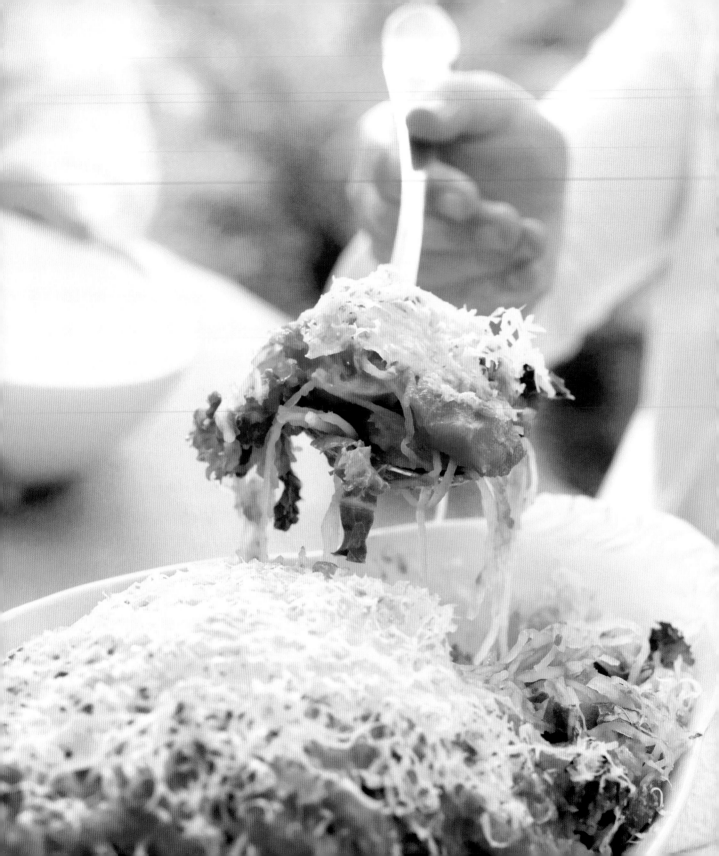

Oh, My! SPAGHETTI SURPRISE

BAKED SPAGHETTI SQUASH WITH CHICKEN SAUSAGE

This recipe is fun to make with kids because they're amazed by how the solid squash magically becomes thin strands of "spaghetti" after it's cooked! This fun factor also makes them more likely to try the dish once the squash is mixed with bone-building kale, juicy tomatoes and flavorful chicken sausage. You'll be happy knowing just one serving delivered 70 percent of a day's worth of vitamin A, 80 percent of the daily requirement for vitamin C and nearly 20 percent of the minerals iron and calcium.

YIELD: 6 servings | **TIME:** 50 minutes

1 small spaghetti squash, halved lengthwise and seeded

2 tbsp/30 ml vegetable oil

½ cup/8 g finely chopped onion

4 cloves garlic, finely chopped

1 ½ tsp/1.4 g thyme leaves

1 tbsp/20 g tomato paste

1 (28 oz/784 g) can whole tomatoes

4 oz/112 g Tuscan kale, sliced in ½"/1.3 cm strips, tough stems removed

12 oz/340 g precooked chicken sausage, sliced

6 tbsp/30 g finely grated Parmigiano-Reggiano

Preheat oven to 350°F/180°C or gas mark 4. Place the spaghetti squash on a baking tray with ¼ inch/6 millimeters water, cut side down, and bake until a knife goes in easily, about 30 minutes to an hour depending on size. When cool enough to handle, use a fork, scraping lengthwise, to create the "spaghetti" and scrape into a bowl. Measure 3 cups/765 grams and place in a large bowl. Save the remainder for another use.

While the spaghetti squash is cooking, make tomato sauce. Place a large saucepan over medium heat. Add the vegetable oil and sauté the onion until golden, 2 minutes. Add the garlic and thyme and cook until aromatic, another 30 seconds. Add the tomato paste and stir to allow the tomato paste to caramelize, about 1 minute. Add the canned tomatoes and simmer the sauce for 10 minutes.

Place a large pot of salted water over high heat and bring to a boil. Add the Tuscan kale and simmer until tender, about 5 minutes, depending on how mature the kale is. Drain the kale. Place in the bowl with the spaghetti squash. Add the chicken sausage and tomato sauce. Toss well and place in a 9 x 13-inch/23 x 33-centimeter baking dish. Sprinkle with the cheese and bake until heated through and cheese is melted, about 15 minutes.

PER SERVING: Calories 250, protein 19 g, total fat 13 g, carbohydrates 19 g, sodium 810 mg, fiber 3 g

TINA'S TIP: Spaghetti squash can be frozen. Place leftovers in zip-top bags, squeeze out air and freeze. Thaw before use. To thaw quickly, place in a bowl of hot water or microwave.

Chow THESE CHOPS

BONELESS PORK CHOPS WITH BEET AND ORANGE RELISH

If you're health-conscious and you're not eating beets, it's time to try this nutrient-packed veggie—and I'm not talking about pickled beets from a can. Beets are a root vegetable, like potatoes, and they're easy to dress up or down. Surprisingly, beets don't need to be cooked; they can be grated and served raw (just don't wear white! Beet juice has a tendency to splatter). You'll love beets knowing they contain folic acid, which helps maintain healthy cells and guards against cancer and heart disease, and they provide fiber, vitamins and powerful antioxidants. Plus, kids will find the magenta hue of these shredded beets appealing because they're eye candy! Bottom line: When it comes to taste and nutrition, you can't beat beets.

YIELD: 4 servings plus 1 ½ cups/105 g slaw | **TIME:** 20 minutes

2 (11 oz/308 g) cans mandarin oranges, well drained

¾ cup/169 g scrubbed, peeled and grated beets

⅓ cup/20 g parsley, chopped

½ tsp salt, divided

4 boneless pork chops, center cut

¼ tsp pepper

½ tbsp/7.5 ml canola oil

In a medium bowl, add oranges, beets, parsley and ¼ teaspoon of the salt, stirring to combine. Season pork chops with remaining ¼ teaspoon salt and pepper. In a large sauté pan over high heat, warm oil. Add seasoned pork chops, and lower the heat to medium-high. Sauté until pork chops are golden brown on each side and cooked in the center, about 4 minutes per side. Serve pork chops topped with relish.

PER SERVING: Calories 230, protein 26 g, total fat 10 g, carbohydrates 9 g, sodium 380 mg, fiber 1 g

TINA'S TIP: For a different variation, try chopped mint instead of parsley. It adds a bright, fresh flavor!

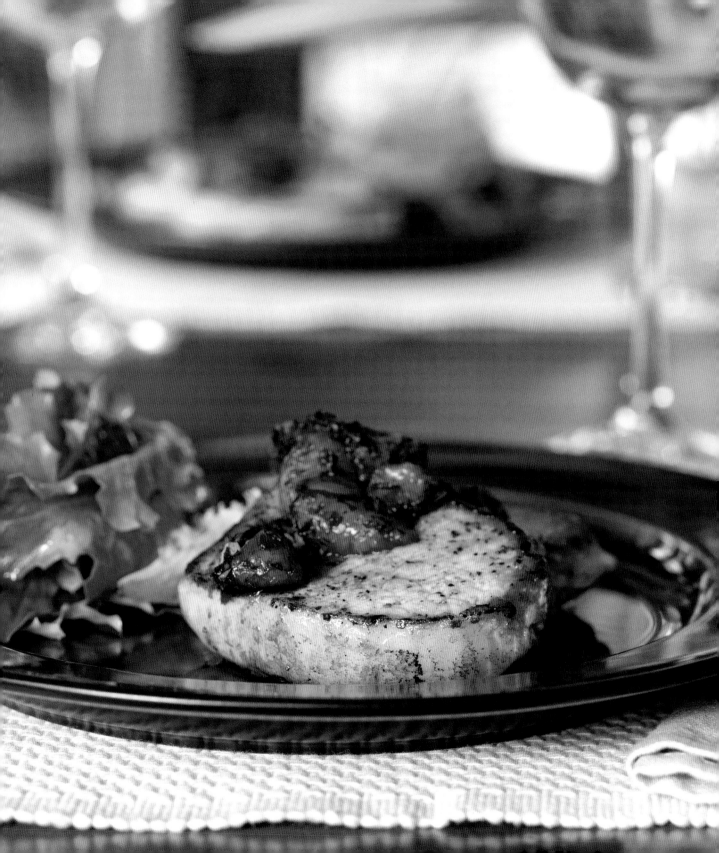

Simply SAVORY STUFFED PORK

STUFFED PORK LOIN WITH SWISS CHARD, ROASTED RED PEPPER, PINE NUTS AND RAISINS

On Sunday, when everyone is preoccupied with homework, watching television or tackling chores, I like to cook a big meal, enough to make leftovers for the coming week. If this sounds like you, you'll love my stuffed pork. It looks impressive yet takes very little skill. Pork tenderloin is an excellent source of protein and, ounce for ounce, has less fat than a chicken breast. The Swiss chard contributes vitamins A, C, K and fiber, and each serving is a good source of B vitamins, minerals, zinc and phosphorous.

YIELD: 12 servings | **TIME:** 1 hour 30 minutes

3 tbsp/45 ml vegetable oil, divided

1 shallot, finely chopped

3 cloves garlic, finely chopped

½ tsp fresh thyme leaves

4 leaves Swiss chard, finely sliced

Salt and pepper

1 roasted red pepper, finely chopped

2 tbsp/18 g pine nuts, roughly chopped

¼ cup/36 g raisins, roughly chopped

¼ cup/30 g breadcrumbs

1 oz/28 g Parmigiano-Reggiano, finely grated

1 egg

3 lb/1,365 g pork loin, butterflied for stuffing and rolling

Preheat oven to 375°F/190°C, or gas mark 5. Heat a large sauté pan over medium-high heat. Add 1 tablespoon/15 milliliters of the vegetable oil and the shallot. Sauté until golden, about 5 minutes, then add the garlic and thyme. Cook an additional 30 seconds, until aromatic. Add the Swiss chard and cook until softened, about 3 minutes. If the Swiss chard is tough, add a splash of water to the pan to soften it. Season with salt and pepper.

Transfer the Swiss chard mixture to a bowl and add the roasted red pepper, pine nuts, raisins, breadcrumbs and Parmigiano-Reggiano. Taste the mixture and adjust seasoning with salt and pepper. Stir in the egg.

Unroll the pork loin. Season the inside with salt and pepper. Spread the filling across the pork loin. Roll the pork loin back up and place the seam side down. Using butcher's twine, tie the pork at 2-inch/5-centimiter intervals. Season the outside with salt and pepper.

Heat a large ovenproof sauté pan over medium-high heat. Add the remaining 2 tablespoons/30 milliliters vegetable oil to coat the bottom of the pan. Place the pork loin in the pan and brown on all sides. Transfer the pan to the oven and cook until an instant-read thermometer reads 150°F/65°C, approximately 50 to 55 minutes. Let cool for 10 minutes before slicing.

PER SERVING: Calories 156, protein 24 g, total fat 16 g, carbohydrates 8 g, sodium 530 mg, fiber 1 g

TINA'S TIP: If you don't have raisins and Swiss chard, play with different dried fruits such as apricots or other hearty greens like kale or collards or even spinach in a pinch.

Homemade **HOLIDAY HIT**

SEARED PEPPERED BEEF TENDERLOIN, MUSHROOMS AND CRANBERRY PAN SAUCE

Everyone should have a special-occasion recipe in his or her back pocket, and this is one of my favorites. It can be made quickly with a few simple ingredients and produces great results time and again. When you have confidence in a recipe, cooking for company becomes enjoyable, and you can spend more time with your guests and less time in the kitchen. When you cook with wine, you don't have to use an expensive bottle, just a wine you'd be willing to drink. Stay away from anything labeled "cooking wine," which tastes horrible and is likely filled with flavorings, preservatives and sodium. Feel free to double this recipe for a bigger group, and it will turn out perfectly!

YIELD: 4 servings | **TIME:** 20 minutes

4 (4 oz/112 g) portions beef tenderloin

Salt to taste

1 tsp/2 g coarsely ground black pepper, or more to taste

1 tbsp/15 ml vegetable oil, divided

¼ cup/40 g finely chopped shallots

½ tsp thyme leaves

¾ cup/60 g finely chopped cremini mushrooms

½ cup/120 ml red wine

¼ cup/36 g dried cranberries, preferably no sugar added

1 cup/240 ml low-sodium beef stock

1 tbsp/4 g parsley, finely chopped

Preheat oven to 400°F/200°C or gas mark 6. Heat a sauté pan over medium-high heat. Season the steaks with salt and black pepper. Add 2 teaspoons/10 milliliters of the oil to the pan and brown steaks on both sides, about 2 minutes per side. Transfer steaks to a baking tray and place in the oven. Cook for 8 minutes for medium-rare. Let the meat rest for 5 minutes before serving. Any juices that accumulate should be added to the pan sauce.

While the steaks are cooking, make the pan sauce. Reduce heat to medium-low. Add the remaining 1 teaspoon/5 milliliters oil to the pan along with the shallots, thyme and mushrooms. Sprinkle with a little salt. Cook until shallots and mushrooms are softened and starting to brown and thyme is aromatic, about 2 minutes. Deglaze the pan with the red wine, whisking to scrape up all the flavorful brown bits along the bottom of the pan. Add the cranberries. Increase heat to bring wine to a boil and reduce by half, about 3 minutes. Add the beef stock. Bring to a boil and reduce by about half, 5 minutes. Taste and adjust seasonings. Stir in parsley. Place each piece of tenderloin on a serving plate and top with sauce.

PER SERVING: Calories 210, protein 24 g, total fat 8 g, carbohydrates 9 g, sodium 280 mg, fiber 0 g

TINA'S TIP: When you're hosting a dinner party, you can brown the steak and move it to the baking tray, covered loosely with foil, and it will keep for up to an hour. In the meanwhile, you can make the sauce and reserve it until needed. When ready, just pop the steaks in the oven, and you're set!

Make **MY MEATBALLS**

APRICOT-STUDDED MINI MEATBALLS WITH LEMONY COUSCOUS

These little meatballs are so good; I guarantee they'll become a family favorite. Studded with tiny bits of apricots and sprinkled with feta, they make a satisfying dinner without the fuss. Best of all, this dish is a rich source of heart-healthy fats, thanks to the olive oil, and full of bone-building calcium from the feta cheese. Also, it contributes 20 percent of your daily requirements of vitamins A and C and the mineral iron.

YIELD: 16 meatballs, or 4 servings | **TIME:** 30 minutes

1 lb/455 g lean ground beef

¼ cup/33 g finely chopped dried apricots

½ tsp curry powder

1 cup/175 g dry couscous

3 tbsp/45 ml olive oil, plus extra for drizzling

3 tbsp/45 ml lemon juice

Salt and pepper to taste

4 oz/128 g feta cheese, reduced fat

½ cucumber, sliced

1 tomato, sliced

Red onions, sliced (optional)

Preheat broiler. In a large bowl, mix ground beef with apricots and curry powder until well combined. Shape mixture into 16 small meatballs. Place on broiler pan and broil for 6 to 8 minutes, rotating meatballs halfway through the cooking time.

Meanwhile, prepare couscous according to package directions. Whisk together olive oil and lemon juice, seasoning the dressing with salt and pepper. Add dressing to couscous.

To serve, equally divide the couscous among 4 plates. Put 4 meatballs atop each mound of couscous. Sprinkle with feta cheese, and serve accompanied by sliced cucumbers, tomatoes and onions. Pass a little extra olive oil for drizzling.

PER SERVING: Calories 430, total fat 15 g, protein 32 g, carbohydrates 44 g, sodium 200 mg, fiber 7 g

WOK This Way

STIR-FRY OF BEEF, SHIITAKES, BOK CHOY AND SNOW PEAS OVER JASMINE RICE

Beef is a concentrated source of good nutrition, and there are nearly thirty varieties of lean beef to choose from. While the trend today is to go meatless, I prepare beef once or twice a week for my family, knowing they'll get a host of essential minerals, B vitamins and high-quality protein in a very small serving. Choose grass-fed beef for its higher omega-3 fatty acid content, or opt for a lean cut of meat, and braise, roast, marinate or stew to create a mouthwatering, healthy meal. This recipe uses flank steak, a lean cut of beef with lots of flavor. Cook it to medium-rare for best results. One serving delivers 35 percent vitamin A, 20 percent vitamin C and 15 percent iron, and the majority of fat comes from oleic acid, a healthy monounsaturated fat also found in olive oil.

YIELD: 6 servings | **TIME:** 25 minutes

---

1 ½ cups/300 g jasmine rice

5 cups/1,175 ml cold water

12 oz/340 g flank steak

3 tbsp/24 g cornstarch

½ cup/100 g sugar

3 tbsp/45 ml rice vinegar

2 tbsp/30 ml sesame oil

¼ cup/60 ml soy sauce

2 tbsp/30 ml sriracha sauce, or more to taste

2 tbsp/16 g grated ginger

2 tbsp/20 g grated garlic

1 tbsp/15 ml vegetable oil

2 cups/160 g sliced shiitake mushroom caps

4 cups/360 g roughly chopped bok choy

1 cup/100 g snow peas

½ cup/50 g thinly sliced scallion

Place the rice in a saucepan with 3 cups/705 milliliters of the cold water. Bring to a boil, reduce to a simmer, cover and cook for 20 minutes, or until water is absorbed.

While the rice is cooking, prepare the stir-fry. Slice the flank steak by cutting against the grain (flank has distinct "lines" known as the grain) at a 45-degree angle into thin strips (no more than ¼ inch/6 millimeters thick). This helps tenderize the meat. Cut the strips in half. Reserve.

In a large bowl, whisk together the cornstarch, sugar, rice vinegar, sesame oil, soy sauce, sriracha, ginger, garlic and remaining 2 cups/470 milliliters water. Place the steak in the bowl. Let steak marinate for at least 15 minutes while you prepare the vegetables.

Heat a large, heavy sauté pan (preferably at least 12 inches/30 centimeters) over high heat. Remove the steak from the marinade, removing as much liquid as possible, reserving marinade. Add the oil to the pan and carefully lower the meat in to avoid spattering. Use tongs to spread the meat out into one layer. Let it brown, about 1 minute, then start moving it around to get more browning on the other side, 30 seconds. Remove to a bowl. Add the shiitakes and bok choy using the same technique of spreading out the vegetables, initially not moving them to allow some browning, about 1 minute. Add the snow peas, scallions, reserved steak and marinade. Stir together. Sauce will thicken and become clear brown. For each serving, place ½ cup/80 grams rice in a serving bowl and top with about 1 cup/240 grams of the stir-fry mixture.

PER SERVING: Calories 410, protein 15 g, total fat 12 g, carbohydrates 61 g, sodium 300 mg, fiber 2 g

Zorba **THE GREEK**

LAMB BURGERS WITH CUCUMBER GREEK YOGURT SAUCE

I'll be the first to admit that lamb isn't what comes to mind when I want to prepare a family meal, but it deserves consideration for many reasons. Of course, I've made lamb for Easter, but simple, ground lamb is absolutely delicious for any day of the week and an excellent source of high-quality protein, B vitamins, iron, zinc and selenium. Certified organic lamb is available, if you want to go that route, but no matter whether the lamb you buy is organic or not, it will be a source of omega-3 fatty acids, conjugated linoleic acid (CLA), which has been shown to lower the risk of heart disease, and tryptophan, which can help regulate appetite and improve sleep. I like to make this dish on summer weekends when we have a barbecue. It's a wonderful change of pace from hamburgers, but just as simple to make, and everyone loves it. The cucumber-yogurt sauce is cooling and refreshing, and combined, the meal is absolutely yummy.

YIELD: 4 burgers | **TIME:** 30 minutes

1 lb/455 g ground lamb

2 tsp/6 g grated garlic

1 tsp/2.5 g (plus a pinch for yogurt sauce) ground cumin

2 tsp/5 g ground coriander

¼ cup/15 g parsley, roughly chopped

2 tsp/10 ml sriracha sauce (optional)

¾ tsp salt plus a pinch

½ tsp freshly ground black pepper plus a pinch

5 tbsp/70 g nonfat Greek yogurt

½ cup/60 g finely chopped or grated cucumber

5 leaves mint, finely chopped

2 tsp/10 ml vegetable oil

4 burger buns

4 leaves crisp lettuce such as Boston, romaine or Bibb

4 thick slices beefsteak tomato

Place the lamb, garlic, cumin, coriander, parsley, sriracha, salt and pepper in a bowl. Mix well to combine, making sure there are no pockets of spices that haven't been worked in. Divide the mixture into 4 patties about 4 inches/ 10 centimeters across.

In a separate bowl, combine the yogurt, cucumber, mint, and a pinch each of cumin, salt and pepper. Taste and adjust seasonings. Reserve.

Heat a grill pan or outdoor grill over medium-high heat. Brush the vegetable oil on both sides of the burgers. Place the burgers on the grill and cook until nicely charred and golden brown, about 2 minutes, then flip and repeat on the second side.

Toast the burger buns, if desired. To assemble, place the bottom half of the burger buns on a work surface. Top with 1 lettuce leaf, 1 slice of tomato, a burger and one-fourth of the yogurt sauce. Top with other half of bun.

PER BURGER: Calories 320, protein 23 g, total fat 18 g, carbohydrates 17 g, sodium 500 mg, fiber 3 g

TINA'S TIP: Try making these into skewers: make 1-inch/2.5-centimeter balls of the lamb mixture, then roll them into a cylinder. Skewer and grill. Serve the yogurt sauce as a dipping sauce. You'll be the hit of any barbecue!

DESERT Song

MOROCCAN CHICKEN TAGINE WITH DRIED FRUIT

Chicken is like a fashion model; unadorned, it's rather plain, but dressed up it'll knock your socks off! This recipe illustrates my point. I use rather unglamorous chicken thighs, but with the addition of herbs, dried fruit and seasonings, you have a high-impact meal that's hard to forget. As for my choice of dark meat, I prefer it because it has a richer taste and more succulent texture. White meat has fewer calories and fat than dark meat, but the darker meat has much more nutrition, including B vitamins, iron and zinc.

YIELD: 4 servings | **TIME:** 1 hour

4 (4 oz/112 g) skinless, bone-in chicken thighs

Salt and pepper

2 tsp/10 ml vegetable oil

1 cup/160 g diced onion

4 cloves garlic, roughly chopped

2 tbsp/8 g grated ginger

1 tsp/5 ml sriracha or hot sauce (optional)

1 tbsp/7 g cumin

1 tbsp/7 g coriander

½ tsp cinnamon

2 carrots, sliced

1 quart/940 ml low-sodium chicken stock

1 cup/165 g roughly chopped dried apricots (or prunes, raisins, dates, cranberries or cherries, or a combination of mixed, dried fruit)

½ cup/8 g cilantro, roughly chopped

½ cup/50 g thinly sliced scallions (optional)

Whole wheat couscous, for serving

Heat a Dutch oven or large soup pot over medium heat. Season chicken with salt and pepper. Add enough oil to coat the bottom of the pan and brown the chicken on both sides. Add the onion and cook until starting to brown, about 5 minutes. Add the garlic, ginger, sriracha, cumin, coriander and cinnamon and cook until aromatic, about 1 minute. Add the carrots, stock and dried fruit. Bring to a simmer and cook for 30 minutes. Chicken should be tender and falling off the bone. Taste and adjust seasonings. Remove from heat and sprinkle with cilantro and scallions. Serve atop a generous serving of fluffy couscous. Like any stew, this will taste even better if it has more time to cook or if it's eaten the next day. This dish will keep for up to 3 days, tightly covered, in the refrigerator.

PER SERVING: Calories 300, protein 27 g, total fat 8 g, carbohydrates 33 g, sodium 570 mg, fiber 2 g

TINA'S TIP: Sprinkle toasted, slivered almonds over the couscous for added crunch and nutrition.

Hot MAMA

MINI TURKEY MEATLOAF WITH CHIPOTLE GLAZE

These tasty meatloaf minis are mega nutritious, thanks to the oats, sweet potato and lean, ground turkey I've incorporated. Baking them in muffin tins makes them even more irresistible! If you have young children, the adobo sauce can be omitted, but if you're preparing these for teens or adults, absolutely use it. The sauce gives the meatloaf a smoky flavor, and it adds a little kick to the glaze. For a surprising and yummy party appetizer, cut the meatloaf into pieces and serve them warmed on a platter with toothpicks for easy enjoyment! Your guests won't even know the dish is healthy, providing 25 percent vitamin A, 15 percent vitamin C and 8 percent iron!

YIELD: 8 mini meatloaves | **TIME:** 30 minutes

1 tbsp/15 ml canola oil

½ cup/80 g chopped onion

2 cups/220 g grated sweet potato (about 1 medium sweet potato)

1 cup/120 g zucchini (about 1 medium zucchini)

1 lb/455 g ground turkey

1 large egg

1 tsp/6 g kosher salt

¼ tsp freshly ground black pepper

¾ cup/60 g quick-cooking oats

2 tsp/10 ml adobo sauce (from 1 can chipotles in adobo)

⅓ cup/80 g ketchup

1 tbsp/15 ml honey

½ tsp adobo sauce

Preheat oven to 350°F/180 or gas mark 4°C.

In a large saucepan, warm oil over medium-high heat. Add onion, sweet potato and zucchini to the pan, stirring and sautéing until the vegetables have softened, about 6 minutes. Remove from heat, and let cool for a few minutes. Meanwhile, in a large bowl, add turkey, egg, salt, pepper, oats and adobo sauce, stirring to combine. Incorporate reserved vegetables into the meat mixture, stirring to combine. Coat an 8-cup muffin tin with cooking spray, and pack meat mixture into each muffin cup. Bake for 10 minutes.

Meanwhile, in a small bowl, combine ketchup, honey and adobo sauce. Top the mini meatloaves with 2 teaspoons/10 milliliters of glaze, and continue to cook 5 additional minutes. Remove from oven, let cool a few minutes and serve. If needed, use a knife to go around the edges of each meatloaf to remove from muffin pan.

PER SERVING: Calories 170, protein 17 g, total fat 4 g, carbohydrates 18 g, sodium 740 mg, fiber 2 g

TINA'S TIP: These mini meatloaves go well with the Yam, Yam Good! on page 138 or with the "Belgian" Slaw on page 129. Use any leftover glaze for meatloaf sandwiches the following day. The glaze will even go well with pork chops!

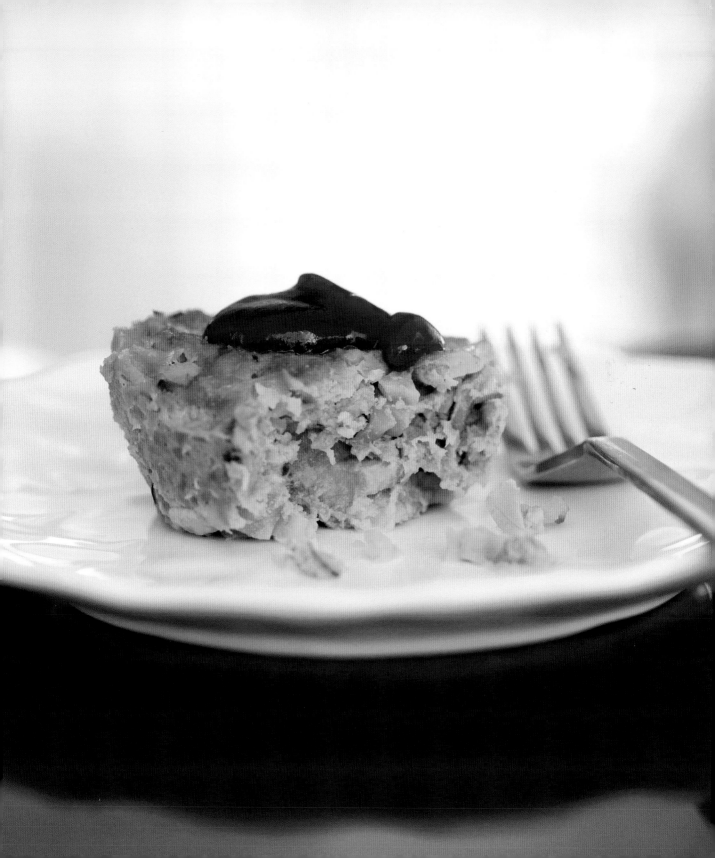

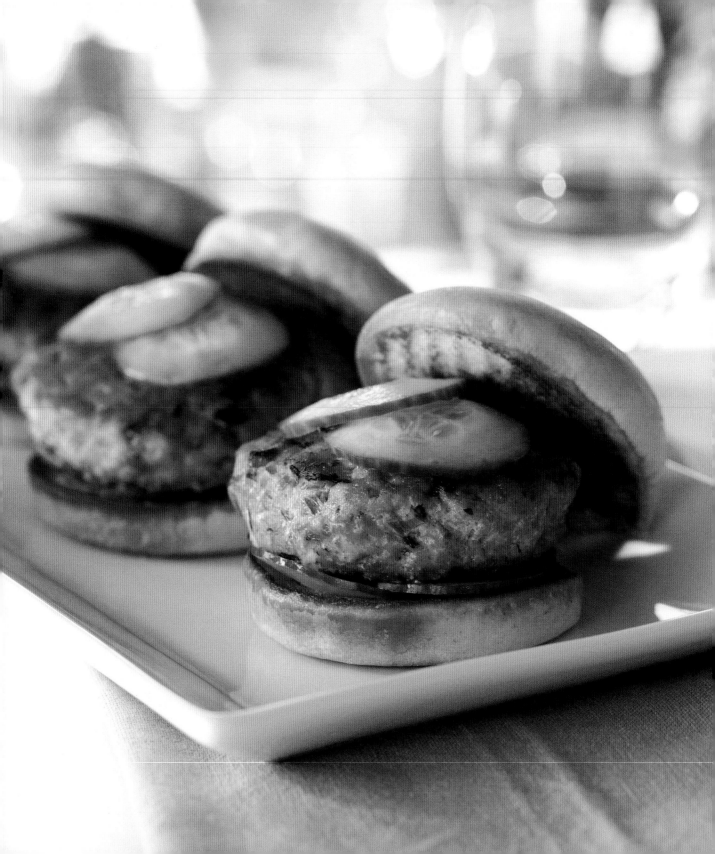

Do the **SALMON SLIDE**

MINI SALMON SLIDERS

We're constantly being exposed to germs, whether at school, the office, the mall or the grocery store. However, a good diet can help keep immunity strong, and loading up on healthy omega-3 fatty acids will do just that. Omega-3s such as EPA and DHA are best absorbed and utilized by the body when the source is seafood. Enjoying 8 to 12 ounces (224 to 336 grams) of cold-water fish weekly is a smart and easy way to stay strong! Studies suggest that 500 mg daily of EPA and DHA are beneficial to health, and just one of these little sliders delivers nearly 600 mg, along with 120 percent of a day's worth of vitamin A along with flavor and fun! They're a great way to get kids enjoying fish for younger children, set aside half the salmon, and prepare it without scallions and curry paste.

YIELD: 12 sliders | **TIME:** 30 minutes

24 oz/680 g Atlantic salmon, cubed

2 tsp/4 g ground coriander

2 tbsp/28 g red curry paste

½ cup/8 g cilantro

½ cup/50 g chopped scallion

2 tbsp/30 ml plus 1 ½ tsp/7.5 ml fish sauce, divided

6 oz/168 g cucumber (preferably hothouse), thinly sliced

¾ tsp rice vinegar

1 tbsp/15 ml vegetable oil

12 silver dollar rolls, dinner rolls or mini hamburger buns

Place the salmon, coriander and red curry paste in the bowl of a food processor fitted with a steel blade. Pulse until well combined, and then add the cilantro, scallion and 2 tablespoons/30 milliliters of the fish sauce. Pulse to incorporate. Form the mixture into 12 patties, approximately 2 ½ inches/ 6.3 centimeters in diameter. Patties can be frozen at this point. Transfer to the refrigerator to defrost before proceeding.

Toss the cucumber with the rice vinegar and remaining 1 ½ teaspoon/ 7.5 milliliters fish sauce. Reserve.

Preheat oven to 200°F/93°C. Heat a nonstick skillet over medium heat. Brush with a little of the vegetable oil. Cook half of the patties until browned on one side, about 2 minutes, then repeat on the second side. Place them on a baking tray in the oven to keep warm. Repeat with the remaining patties. Toast burger buns or rolls, if desired. Place bottoms on a work surface and top with the cucumbers. Top each with a pattie. Drizzle the juices from the cucumber on the top half of each bun before closing.

PER SLIDER: Calories 180, protein 14 g, total fat 7 g, carbohydrates 14 g, sodium 440 mg, fiber 1 g

TINA'S TIP: This recipe can be made with shrimp, too, and it's a great alternative for summertime barbecues. Green or yellow curry pastes will achieve slightly different flavors (and colors) but also work beautifully.

The **THREE MUSKETEERS**

BAKED SALMON WITH BLACKBERRY AND PEAR COMPOTE

Sometimes, the simplest of recipes can be the most impressive, and this is one that will have everyone talking. It's elegant yet easy to prepare, and it makes such a beautiful presentation. The first time I made this dish was when my in-laws came to visit, and it was a hit! I couldn't have been happier (or more relieved). You can even make the compote in advance, and warm it before serving. No matter how you decide to prepare this recipe, you'll enjoy a delicious dinner that's also a rich source of heart-healthy omega-3 fatty acids and antioxidants.

YIELD: 4 servings | **TIME:** 25 minutes

¾ cup/128 g diced pear

½ cup/75 g blackberries

¼ cup/40 g finely diced red onion

1 tsp/4 g sugar

4 (4 oz/112 g) filets wild salmon

Salt and pepper

1 tbsp/4 g parsley, chopped

Preheat oven to 400°F/200°C, or gas mark 6. Place the pear, blackberries, onion and sugar in a small saucepan. Bring to a simmer and cook until heated through and just beginning to soften, about 10 minutes. Reserve.

While the compote is cooking, cook the salmon. Place the salmon on a baking tray and season with a sprinkle of salt and pepper. Place in the oven and cook for 10 minutes for medium-done or longer if desired. Just before serving, stir the parsley into the pear and blackberry compote. Place the salmon on a plate and top with compote.

PER SERVING: Calories 190, protein 23 g, total fat 7 g, carbohydrates 7 g, sodium 50 mg, fiber 2 g

TINA'S TIP: Studies show that those who eat fish twice a week have a longer life expectancy than those who don't. They also have a lower risk of heart disease and less abdominal fat. Try this recipe with Arctic char for a nice change of pace from Alaskan or Norwegian salmon.

The MEATLESS MEDITERRANEAN

BAKED FISH WITH TOMATOES, ONIONS, GARLIC, BASIL, CAPERS AND BREADCRUMBS

When time is tight and everyone is hungry, it's important that I put a meal on the table that's nutritious; I don't believe that a lack of time should compromise the quality of what I serve my family. So, this recipe—a version of a dish my grandmother used to make for me when I was little—is perfect. By the time everyone washes their hands, helps set the table and decides what they want to drink, the fish is done. As for the capers and onions, they can be an acquired taste for younger children, so if you choose to leave them out, the flavor won't be compromised and neither will the nutrition profile. Fish is an incredible source of lean protein, and this recipe provides 45 percent of a day's worth of immune-boosting vitamin C.

YIELD: 4 servings | **TIME:** 25 minutes

1 cup/ 160 g thinly sliced onion

2 tsp/6 g finely chopped garlic

3 cups/540 g roughly chopped tomatoes

½ tsp fresh thyme leaves

¼ cup/10 g basil leaves, sliced

2 tbsp/17 g capers

4 (4 oz/112 g) filets haddock, cod, grouper, red snapper, perch or another fish of uniform thickness

¼ tsp each salt and pepper

¼ cup/30 g breadcrumbs

Preheat oven to 375°F/190°C or gas mark 5. Combine onion, garlic, tomatoes, thyme, basil and capers in a small bowl. Place fish in a baking dish. Sprinkle with ¼ teaspoon salt and pepper to taste. Top with tomato mixture, creating an even layer. Sprinkle with breadcrumbs. Bake for 20 minutes, or until fish is just beginning to flake and/or a knife inserted into the fish is very hot to the touch.

PER SERVING: Calories 180, protein 23 g, total fat 1 g, carbohydrates 17 g, sodium 640 mg, fiber 2 g

TINA'S TIP: This dish goes with just about anything. Serve with a side of brightly colored veggies like broccoli and some whole wheat couscous, brown rice or orzo pasta.

Super SIMPLE SENSATION

FISH EN PAPILLOTE WITH CARROTS, ASPARAGUS, GINGER, GARLIC, SOY SAUCE AND SESAME OIL

You'd never think that three teenage boys would enthusiastically devour salmon en papillote, but I saw it with my own eyes. The fish was gone in minutes, as was the jasmine rice I served on the side. It was the preparation that caught their attention. Cooking anything en papillote just means steaming it in a pouch. That pouch can be foil, banana leaves, parchment or any number of other things. What I like about cooking this way is that you don't need much fat, if any; the steaming preserves the ingredient's nutrition, and you end up with a tender, juicy meal. All this just confirms my theory: new preparation of something familiar can add excitement, satisfaction and nutrition to mealtime.

YIELD: 4 servings | **TIME:** 30 minutes

2 tsp/6 g grated ginger

2 tsp/6 g grated garlic

4 tsp/20 ml soy sauce

1 tsp/5 ml sesame oil

½ tsp sugar

1 cup/130 g julienned carrot

20 pieces pencil asparagus, trimmed of tough stems

8 cherry tomatoes, halved

4 (4 oz/112 g) filets salmon

¼ cup/60 ml white wine

Preheat oven to 400°F/200°C or gas mark 6. Combine the ginger, garlic, soy sauce, sesame oil and sugar in a small bowl. Reserve.

Cut 4 pieces of parchment paper or foil approximately 16 inches/40.5 centimeters long. Fold in half to make a crease to mark the middle of the papers. For each serving, place ¼ cup/33 grams of carrots, 5 pieces of asparagus and 4 cherry tomato halves in the middle of one side. Top with salmon. Spread with one-fourth of the ginger paste and 1 tablespoon/15 milliliters white wine. To close the paper or foil, start at the bottom and make a fold, then continue around the fish. The trick is that with each additional fold you should shape the paper/foil to surround the fish and vegetables and include a portion of the previous fold. On the last fold, tuck the paper/foil under to secure. Place fish on a baking sheet and bake for 10 minutes. Be careful opening up the packets—the steam is hot!

PER SERVING: Calories 230, protein 25 g, total fat 9 g, carbohydrates 10 g, sodium 200 mg, fiber 3 g

TINA'S TIP: Any quick-cooking vegetable can work en papillote as long as it's finely cut. Vegetables with longer cooking times can be par-boiled or blanched. Red-skinned new potatoes, for example, would never cook in the oven in 10 minutes, but boiling them first so they are fork-tender makes them soft and delicious.

FISH IN Paradise

COD WITH AVOCADO AND MANGO SALSA

Fish can be an inexpensive and simple meal to prepare for a family dinner.
I'm especially partial to cod. Snowy white in color, delicate tasting, less expensive
than salmon, tuna and snapper, and caught in the deep, cold waters of the Atlantic,
cod is an incredibly healthy choice that's rich in disease-fighting omega-3 fatty acids.
Topped with this colorful salsa, it's an appealing and satisfying meal. I know firsthand,
because it was lapped up by a group of very hungry college boys!

YIELD: 4 servings | **TIME:** 30 minutes

¾ cup/131 g diced mango

½ cup/90 g diced tomato

½ cup/74 g diced Haas avocado

½ cup/80 g finely chopped red onion (optional)

1 tsp/3 g finely chopped garlic

⅓ cup/5 g cilantro, roughly chopped

1 tbsp/15 ml lime juice

½ tsp sriracha sauce or hot sauce

½ tsp salt, divided

4 (4 oz/112 g) filets cod

1 tsp/5 ml vegetable oil

Place the mango, tomato, avocado, red onion, garlic, cilantro, lime juice, sriracha and ¼ teaspoon of the salt in a bowl. Allow the flavors to meld as the cod is cooked.

Heat a grill pan over medium-high heat. Sprinkle the cod with the remaining ¼ teaspoon salt and brush with the oil. Grill the fish for 3 minutes per side, or until cooked through. To serve, place fish on a serving plate and top with ½ cup/125 g salsa.

PER SERVING: Calories 160, protein 21 g, total fat 4 g, carbohydrates 9 g, sodium 360 mg, fiber 2 g

TINA'S TIP: For a delicious variation, substitute the tomato with cucumber and the cilantro with dill.

Easy Breezy
ISLAND TACOS

SHRIMP TACOS WITH TROPICAL SLAW

On game day, I like to serve lean, healthy meals like these shrimp tacos, because no one does much more than sit on the sofa. I transformed the classic, crispy fish taco into something that's just as fun to eat but far more nutritious. Bean sprouts add vitamin C, cilantro is a natural cleansing agent and red onions contribute the brain-boosting flavonol called quercetin. This recipe is also a perfect example of how simply seasoned, fresh ingredients can taste spectacular. And, who doesn't love to make tacos? It's a great family activity, and I believe it's that camaraderie that keeps everyone together at the table.

YIELD: 8 tacos | **TIME:** 25 minutes

1½ tbsp/22.5 ml sesame oil

1 tbsp/15 ml white vinegar or rice vinegar

½ tbsp/7.5 ml honey

½ tsp salt, divided

4 oz/128 g bean sprouts

1 cup/110 g grated carrot

2 tbsp/20 g finely chopped red onion

½ cup/8 g cilantro, chopped

1¼ lb/569 g large shrimp, peeled and deveined

1 tsp/2 g sweet paprika

¼ tsp pepper

1 tbsp/15 ml canola oil

8 small wheat tortillas

In a medium bowl, whisk together sesame oil, vinegar, honey and ¼ teaspoon of the salt. Add bean sprouts, carrot, onion and cilantro, stirring to combine.

Meanwhile, sprinkle shrimp with paprika, remaining ¼ teaspoon salt and pepper, using your hands to coat shrimp with spices. In a large nonstick sauté pan, warm canola oil over high heat. Add shrimp, stirring and sautéing until shrimp are cooked, about 4 to 5 minutes. Transfer shrimp to a platter alongside slaw and tortillas. Let everyone assemble his or her own tacos to serve.

PER TACO: Calories 210, protein 19 g, total fat 7 g, carbohydrates 17 g, sodium 390 mg, fiber 2 g

TINA'S TIP: If you're not a fan of cilantro, parsley can be subbed instead.

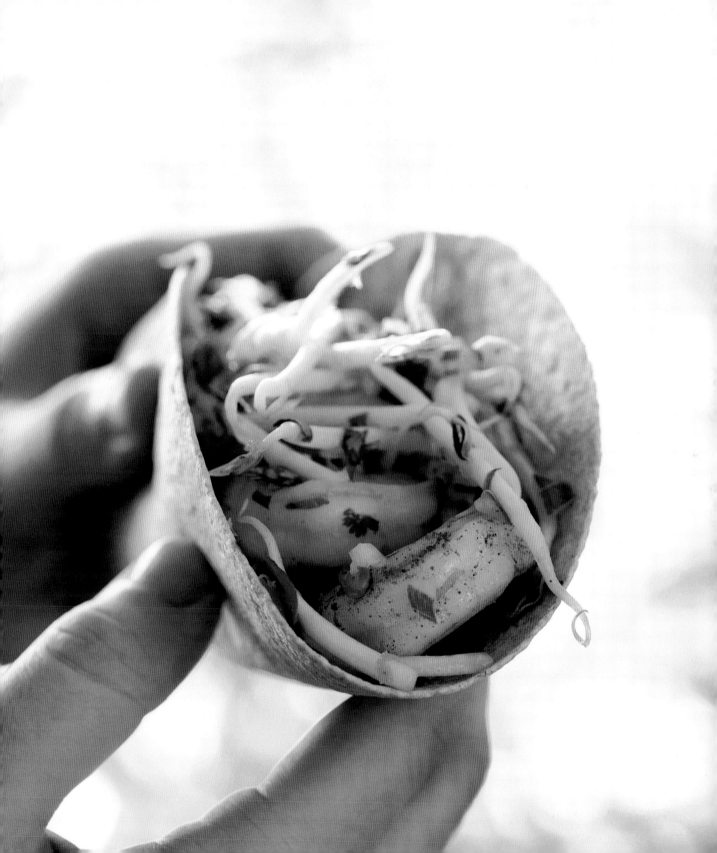

Charming CHARMOULA

HADDOCK WITH FRESH HERB SAUCE

Charmoula is an aromatic marinade popular in Morocco, Algeria and Tunisia. It will jazz up baked and grilled fish or lamb or roasted vegetables. You can even treat it like pesto, mixing it with couscous, rice or roasted potatoes! Cilantro and parsley give the sauce its rich, herbal flavor and gorgeous color along with a healthy dose of antioxidants. Paprika, also added for color and flavor, contributes vitamin C and aids digestion. If you can't find haddock, this recipe is delicious with cod, grouper or sea bass.

YIELD: 4 servings | **TIME:** 30 minutes

¼ cup/4 g cilantro (leaves and stems), roughly chopped

¾ cup/45 g flat-leaf parsley, roughly chopped

4 cloves garlic, roughly chopped

3 tbsp/45 ml lemon juice

1 ½ tsp/3.7 g paprika

½ tsp salt

1 ½ tsp/3.7 g ground cumin

1 tbsp/15 ml extra-virgin olive oil

1 very large beefsteak tomato, sliced into 4 thick slices

4 (4 oz/112 g) filets haddock

Preheat oven to 400°F/200°C, or gas mark 6. To make the charmoula sauce, place the cilantro, parsley, garlic, lemon juice, paprika, salt and cumin in a blender, and purée until smooth. With the motor running, drizzle in the olive oil.

Place the 4 tomato slices along the bottom of a 9 x 9-inch/23 x 23-centimeter pan. Top each tomato with a piece of haddock. Pour the charmoula sauce over the fish and bake until the fish is cooked through, 15 to 20 minutes. Serve each piece of fish with the tomato and charmoula sauce.

PER SERVING: Calories 150, protein 22 g, total fat 4.5 g, carbohydrates 5 g, sodium 380 mg, fiber 1 g

TINA'S TIP: Serve this dish with a side of golden raisin–studded couscous, or simply sauté onions and peppers; it's a classic accompaniment that everyone enjoys!

Spin the **WHEEL**

ROULADE OF COD STUFFED WITH LEEKS, MUSHROOMS AND SPINACH

When I sat down to write this book, I thought long and hard about what defines a family and what constitutes a family meal. Family meals are what you're proud to serve to those you love and at the end of the day, what matters is that you gather to share nourishment and quality time with those who mean the most to you. So, tonight, sit down to my delicious stuffed cod. No matter whether you're serving two or four, this simply healthy meal will make everyone smile, foster good times and inspire memories.

YIELD: 4 servings | **TIME:** 35 minutes

1 tbsp/14 g butter

2 cups/210 g sliced leeks (white and light green parts only)

2 cups/140 g sliced cremini mushrooms

1 tsp thyme leaves, divided

Salt and pepper

6 tbsp/90 ml white wine, divided

3 cups/90 g roughly chopped young leaf spinach

1 lb/454 g cod fillet

1 tbsp/15 ml extra-virgin olive oil

Preheat the oven to 375°F/190°C or gas mark 5. Heat a sauté pan over medium heat. Melt the butter and sauté the leeks until softened but not browned, about 5 minutes. Add the mushrooms and ½ teaspoon of the thyme leaves. Sprinkle with salt and pepper. Continue to cook until the mushrooms have lightly browned and softened, about 5 minutes. Deglaze the pan with 2 tablespoons/30 milliliters of the wine. Add the spinach, cover and cook until wilted, about 2 minutes. Stir the mixture together and adjust the seasoning with salt and pepper to taste. Reserve.

Place the cod on a cutting board and, using a sharp knife, butterfly the fillet, leaving a 1-inch/2.5-centimeter hinge. Open the cod and spread the reserved filling along the fish. Using butcher twine, tie the cod in 3-inch/7.5-centimeter increments. Place the cod on a baking tray. Sprinkle with the remaining ½ teaspoon thyme and the olive oil. Pour the remaining 4 tablespoons/60 milliliters wine over the fish. Place in the oven and bake until cooked through, 10 to 15 minutes.

PER SERVING: Calories 190, protein 22 g, total fat 7 g, carbohydrates 8 g, sodium 100 mg, fiber 2 g

TINA'S TIP: Leeks are notoriously full of sandy dirt. The easiest way to clean them is to cut the leeks lengthwise (white and light green parts only—save the dark green for stock!), then across into ¼-inch/6-millimeter slices. Place them in a large bowl of water to ensure that the dirt can fall to the bottom of the bowl. Pull the leeks out—don't pour the water and leeks into a colander or the dirt will be poured right back onto the leeks!

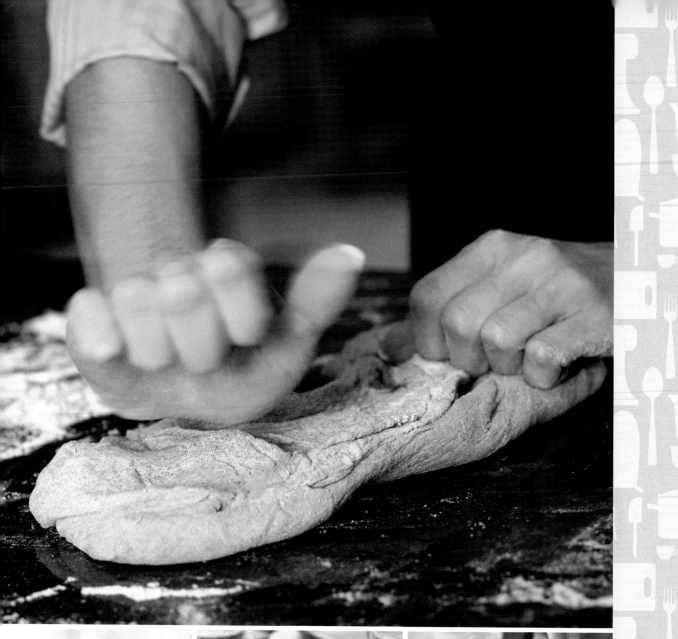

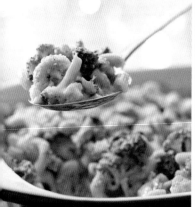

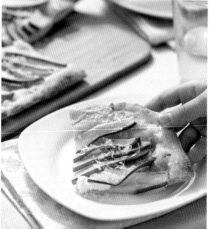

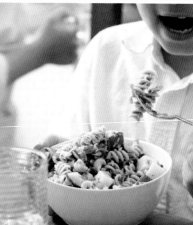

Tempting Pasta, Flatbread and One-Dish Wonders

Simple, filling recipes that will satisfy the biggest appetites while keeping calories in check!

The ageless, iconic Italian screen goddess Sophia Loren once said, "Everything you see, I owe to spaghetti!" Looking at her radiant skin, voluptuous mane of hair and phenomenal figure, I don't think anyone would doubt her.

Pasta is the key to enduring beauty and longevity. Certainly, genetics play a role, which Ms. Loren seemed to dismiss, but pasta is a "good for you food" that I always include in my family's meals.

Since I was a child, I've eaten pasta nearly every evening. It was the primi piatti, or first course, served before our main dish, but the portion size was very small, perhaps a cup. Sometimes, the primi piatti would be soup or risotto, depending upon the season, but needless to say, carbohydrates were featured prominently at the table. Both my grandmother and my mother incorporated whole wheat and traditional pasta into their menus, and we always enjoyed it with light sauces, fresh vegetables or simply a splash of the best-quality olive oil they could find.

Today, with everyone going gluten-free or low carb, they're missing out on taste, health and the ultimate satisfaction that comes from eating something truly satiating. I always tell my family, "Eat something satisfying and you won't be snacking later." And it's true.

Pasta, when prepared properly and eaten in small portions, has the power to effectively fuel activity. When I want my family to perform their best—whether on the ball field or in the classroom—complex carbs are my choice.

Homemade pizza, in addition to the simple and savory one-dish meals I've incorporated into this chapter, can also be a super source of nutrients, so give it a try. You may just find it is the easiest, healthiest and most memorable meal you've brought to your table!

Beyond **BELIEF**

VEGETARIAN CHILI

I'm often asked to bring "one of my delicious entrées" to a potluck—with the reminder that some of the guests are vegan, allergic to nuts, following a gluten-free diet or watching their weight. Coming up with a recipe to accommodate so many diverse requirements has always been a challenge, but this dish is one of my favorites and has never let me down. Contrary to popular belief, tofu and tempeh are not interchangeable, even though they're both made from soybeans. Tempeh has a firm, chewy texture, while tofu is soft and spongy, and tempeh has more protein, making it a more suitable meat alternative.

YIELD: 8 servings | **TIME:** 1 hour

2 tbsp/30 ml vegetable oil

3 cups/480 g roughly chopped onion

4 cloves garlic, finely chopped

1 tbsp/15 g tomato paste

2 tbsp/10 g ground mild chiles (such as New Mexico) or mild chili powder

1 tbsp/5 g ground cumin

¼ tsp salt

1 cup/150 g diced red bell pepper

1 cup/150 g diced green bell pepper

1 cup/120 g diced zucchini

2 bay leaves

1 (28 oz/784 g) can plum tomatoes

1 tbsp/10 g puréed chipotles in adobo, or more to taste

1 (15 oz/420 g) can black beans, rinsed and drained

1 (15 oz/420 g) can chickpeas, rinsed and drained

2 (8 oz/224 g) packages tempeh, cut into 1"/2.5 cm cubes

½ cup/8 g cilantro (leaves and stems), chopped, plus additional for sprinkling

2 cups/470 ml water

Heat a large pot over medium-high heat. Add the oil and sauté the onions until lightly browned, about 5 minutes. Add the garlic, tomato paste, ground chiles, cumin and salt. Stir constantly until aromatic and the tomato paste caramelizes, about 5 minutes. Add the red and green peppers and zucchini and soften, about 2 minutes. Add the bay leaves, tomatoes, puréed chipotles in adobo, black beans, chickpeas, tempeh, cilantro and water. Bring to a simmer, reduce heat and cook for 20 minutes to allow the flavors to meld. Adjust seasoning if needed. Serve 1 ½ cups/300 grams of chili in bowls and sprinkle with additional cilantro.

PER SERVING: Calories 280, protein 18 g, total fat 11 g, carbohydrates 32 g, sodium 105 mg, fiber 8 g

TINA'S TIP: As with any stew, this is even better the next day. Try serving it over toasted quinoa instead of rice, for those who may want a gluten-free option. Otherwise, brown rice is the perfect complement to this dish!

Autumn **HARVEST PASTA**

PASTA WITH BRUSSELS SPROUTS AND RED AND GOLDEN BEETS

If you want to be smart and fit, and you want your children to be the same, then serve pasta. It's a great source of carbohydrates, the brain's and body's most vital energy source. One cup/140 grams of cooked pasta has about 220 calories, a mere gram of fat and no cholesterol. If you prefer to go the whole-grain route, you'll find the same amount of calories as in regular pasta, but a little more protein, fiber and vitamins. No matter which pasta you choose, I promise this recipe will become one of your favorites. The ingredients are humble, but the flavors are extraordinary, the colors vibrant and the aroma mouthwatering. Just one serving offers half a day's worth of vitamin C, 20 percent of your daily need for vitamin A and 15 percent of your iron requirement. What more could you possibly ask for?

YIELD: 4 servings   **TIME:** 50 minutes

---

4 oz/112 g baby red beets, tops removed

6 oz/170 g Brussels sprouts, trimmed and cut into quarters

8 oz/224 g farfalle or other small pasta

¼ cup/56 g unsalted butter

4 cloves garlic, roughly chopped

½ tsp fennel seeds, finely chopped

2 tsp/3.5 g sliced sage leaves

2 tbsp/30 ml white wine

Salt and freshly ground pepper

¼ cup/56 g part-skim ricotta

4 tsp/4 g parsley, roughly chopped, for garnish

Place beets in a pot of salted water. Cover and bring to a boil over high heat; cook until a knife goes into the beets easily, about 30 minutes. Drain. Cool quickly by placing beets in a pot of cold water. Drain when cool, and peel by simply pushing the skins with your fingertips. Cut into bite-size pieces.

While the beets are cooking, bring a large pot of salted water to a boil. Cook the Brussels sprouts until softened, about 5 minutes. Remove the Brussels sprouts from the water and drain. Use the same water to cook the farfalle to al dente, following the package directions, about 11 minutes. Drain and reserve.

Heat a large sauté pan over medium heat. Add the butter. The butter will melt and foam and then begin to brown. Keep an eye on it so that it doesn't burn. When it's brown, add the beets and Brussels sprouts and sauté them until crisp and brown, about 2 minutes. Add the garlic, fennel and sage and cook until aromatic, about 30 seconds. Deglaze the pan with the wine. Cook for another minute, or until most of the wine has been absorbed. Stir in the pasta. Adjust the seasoning with salt and pepper.

Divide the pasta among 4 bowls. Top each bowl with 1 tablespoon/14 grams ricotta and 1 teaspoon/1 gram parsley.

PER SERVING: Calories 350, protein 12 g, total fat 13 g, carbohydrates 53 g, sodium 75 mg, fiber 4 g

TINA'S TIP: If you can find golden beets at the market, mix them with red beets for a dramatic presentation.

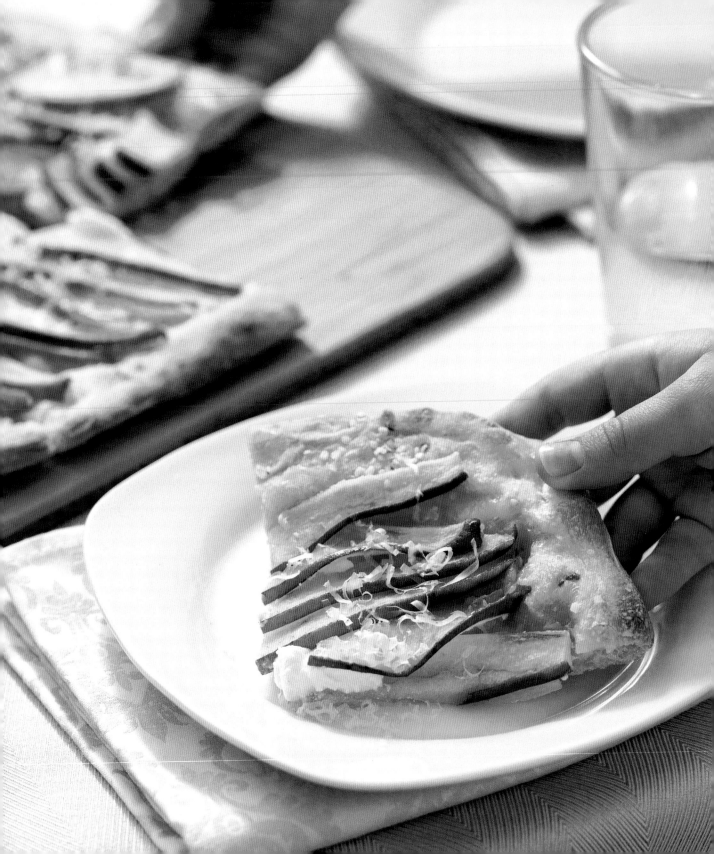

THREE TIMES the Charm

THREE CHEESE FLATBREAD WITH PEARS AND MAPLE DRIZZLE

I find that introducing new ingredients to children—and even adults—is best accomplished when the portions are small or the meal is presented in a familiar way. Fresh pears may seem boring to a child, but atop a crispy pizza crust bubbling with cheese ... success! This recipe is an all-around winner, and the flavor combination is unbeatable. Bosc pears are ideal for baking and go well with cheese. But what's with the hemp seed and maple syrup? Hemp seed provides a punch of protein and the maple rounds out the flavor of this wonderful pie.

YIELD: 8 slices | **TIME:** 35 minutes

Flour, as needed

1 lb/455 g pizza dough, at room temperature

2 tbsp/16 g hemp seed

1½ tbsp/7.5 g finely grated Parmigiano-Reggiano

1 oz/28 g mozzarella, grated

2 tbsp/36 g ricotta cheese

3 medium pears, preferable Bosc

½ tbsp/7.5 ml lemon juice

½ tbsp/7.5 ml maple syrup

Preheat oven to 450°F/230°C or gas mark 8.

Layer a rimmed 16 x 12-inch/40 x 30-centimeter baking sheet with foil and coat with cooking spray. Sprinkle 1 to 2 tablespoons/8 to 16 grams of flour onto a cutting board, and dust both sides of pizza dough with flour. Slowly, stretch the dough on the back of your knuckles, rotating the dough and stretching it out into a rectangular shape to fit the baking sheet. When the dough is stretched out to about 12 inches/30 centimeters, place on the baking sheet and stretch the pizza dough further using your fingertips.

In a small bowl, combine hemp seed and Parmigiano-Reggiano cheese. Sprinkle mixture over the dough, pushing the mixture into the dough. Top mozzarella cheese over the dough, and then dot with ricotta cheese. Trim the stem from each pear and cut each one in half, using a spoon to core each half. Thinly slice each pear and place on dough in 4 vertical layers (as close together as possible), pressing pears into the dough. Drizzle pears with lemon juice and maple syrup. Bake until flatbread is golden brown and pears are cooked, about 15 to 20 minutes. Remove from oven, and let cool slightly. Cut into 8 pieces, and serve.

PER SLICE: Calories: 210, protein 7 g, total fat 5 g, carbohydrates 38 g, sodium 240 mg, fiber 3 g

TINA'S TIP: Let the dough sit at room temperature for an hour or two; the longer it sits, the easier it is to mold into shape. Also, for a grown-up spin on this kid-friendly flatbread, mix ¼ teaspoon to ½ teaspoon of cayenne pepper with the lemon juice to drizzle on pears.

Power **PESTO**

KALE AND PUMPKIN SEED PESTO

When I don't have much time to make dinner, I cook pasta. I also keep a stash of different sauces on hand, so whipping up a truly healthy meal is easy. This pesto is one of my secret sauces. It tastes incredible, freezes beautifully and defrosts in minutes. Besides its convenience, it's also a great source of nutrition. Anchovies deliver protein and calcium, olive oil contributes heart-healthy fat, pumpkin seeds are a concentrated source of fiber and vitamins, and kale is king, when it comes to greens. An unlikely combination for pesto sauce, you say? Of course! But therein is the reason you bought this book; expect your family to love the unexpected, and be healthier because of it.

YIELD: 2 cups/520 g pesto | **TIME:** 25 minutes

4 cups/268 g kale leaves, tough ribs removed

1 cup/40 g basil leaves, tightly packed

2 oz/56 g pumpkin seeds

½ cup/50 g grated Parmigiano-Reggiano

4 cloves garlic

1 tbsp/15 ml lemon juice

6 anchovy filets, rinsed of excess oil and salt

¼ tsp red pepper flakes

½ cup/120 ml extra-virgin olive oil

¼ cup/60 ml warm water

Bring a saucepan of salted water to a boil over high heat. Cook the kale until softened, about 5 minutes. Drain and cool. Place the cooked kale, basil, pumpkin seeds, cheese, garlic, lemon juice, anchovies and red pepper flakes in the bowl of a food processor or blender. Blend to combine. With the motor running, drizzle in the oil and water. Process until a fine paste forms. Pesto can be frozen for up to 3 months.

To serve, toss 2 tablespoons/30 grams of pesto for every ½ cup/70 grams of cooked penne.

PER 2-TABLESPOON/30-GRAM SERVING OF PESTO: Calories 110, protein 3 g, total fat 10 g, carbohydrates 1 g, sodium 120 mg, fiber 0 g

TINA'S TIP: Mustard greens and arugula also make great pesto. They can be substituted for the kale.

Perfect **PUMPKIN SOUP**

BUTTERNUT SQUASH SOUP

Winter squash has an outstanding amount of antioxidant and anti-inflammatory compounds recognized for their cancer-fighting powers, and there's no better way to reap all those benefits than in this velvety soup! What makes it satisfying and healthy is the 1 tablespoon/15 milliliters of cream I add for garnish. The cream makes the vitamin A in the squash more readily absorbed by the body, and it adds a heavenly texture!

YIELD: About 3 quarts/3 liters | **TIME:** 40 minutes plus cooling time

1 tbsp/15 ml vegetable oil

1 medium onion, roughly chopped

4 cloves garlic, smashed

1 small butternut squash, cheese pumpkin or other favorite squash, peeled, seeded and cut into large chunks

Salt and pepper

¾ cup/180 ml heavy cream

Chives, snipped, for garnish (optional)

Heat a large soup pot over medium heat. Add the oil and sauté the onion until softened but not browned, about 10 minutes. Add the garlic and cook until aromatic, about 30 seconds. Add the squash and enough water to cover by 1 inch/2.5 centimeters. Bring to a simmer and cook until soft, about 20 minutes. Season with salt and pepper to taste. Let cool before puréeing in a blender or food processor, or use an immersion blender. To serve, stir 1 tablespoon/15 milliliters cream per 1-cup/235-milliliter portion. Sprinkle with chives.

PER 1–CUP/235–MILLILITER SERVING: Calories 120, protein 2 g, total fat 7 g, carbohydrates 16 g, sodium 10 mg, fiber 3 g

TINA'S TIP: For extra protein, skip the cream, and garnish with a dollop of Greek yogurt and a light dusting of cinnamon. And if you have more soup than you can consume, freeze it! Place the soup in pint containers for small easy-to-thaw batches. Be sure to cool completely before freezing, and leave room for the soup to expand.

Velvety VEGGIE MAC 'N' CHEESE

BROCCOLI-TOMATO BLEND WITH WHOLE WHEAT PENNE AND CHEDDAR CHEESE

Who says mac 'n' cheese can't be part of a healthy diet? New science shows that the protein in cheese can slow the absorption of carbohydrates eaten at the same meal and help keep you full, longer. Even better, this recipe is super simple to make and a real kid-pleaser. It's comforting and flavorful, and you'll be surprised by how little cheese you need to prepare it! A little bit of Parmigiano-Reggiano, an intensely flavored, aged Italian cheese, goes a long way. The result is a colorful, tasty and healthy meal that contributes 35 percent of your day's need for calcium and 30 percent of your vitamin C needs.

YIELD: 8 servings | **TIME:** 30 minutes

---

12 oz/340 g bite-sized broccoli florets

8 oz/224 g whole wheat elbow macaroni

2 tbsp/28 g unsalted butter

1 tsp/3 g finely chopped garlic

3 tbsp/23 g all-purpose flour

2 cups/470 ml low-fat milk

1 cup/100 g grated Parmigiano-Reggiano

½ cup/60 g grated sharp Cheddar cheese

Several grates of nutmeg

Salt and freshly ground pepper

1 ½ cups/240 g large diced tomato

2 tbsp/14 g breadcrumbs

Preheat oven to 350°F/180°C or gas mark 4. Bring a large pot of salted water to a boil over high heat. Cook the broccoli until crisp and tender, about 2 minutes. Remove broccoli (do not drain) and run under cold water to stop the cooking. Use the same water to cook the pasta until al dente according to package directions. Drain pasta and run under cold water to stop the cooking.

Heat a large saucepan over medium-low heat. Add butter and garlic and cook until the garlic is aromatic, 30 seconds. Whisking constantly, stir in the flour, taking care the flour doesn't brown. Continue to cook for 2 minutes. Whisk in the milk. It will thicken as it gets hot. Whisk constantly so any lumps will smooth out. Cook for 5 to 7 minutes, until mixture bubbles and thickens; when it no longer changes in consistency, it's done. Stir in cheeses and nutmeg. Season to taste with salt and pepper. Stir in pasta, broccoli and tomatoes. Spread into a 9 x 9-inch/23 x 23-centimeter pan. Sprinkle with the breadcrumbs. (The dish can be made ahead to this point and refrigerated or frozen.) Bake for 10 minutes, or until heated through.

PER SERVING: Calories 260, protein 15 g, total fat 9 g, carbohydrates 30 g, sodium 420 mg, fiber 2 g

TINA'S TIP: This recipe is incredibly versatile. Start with the basic white sauce, then go to town! Experiment with other small cut pasta, cheeses and different vegetables your family enjoys.

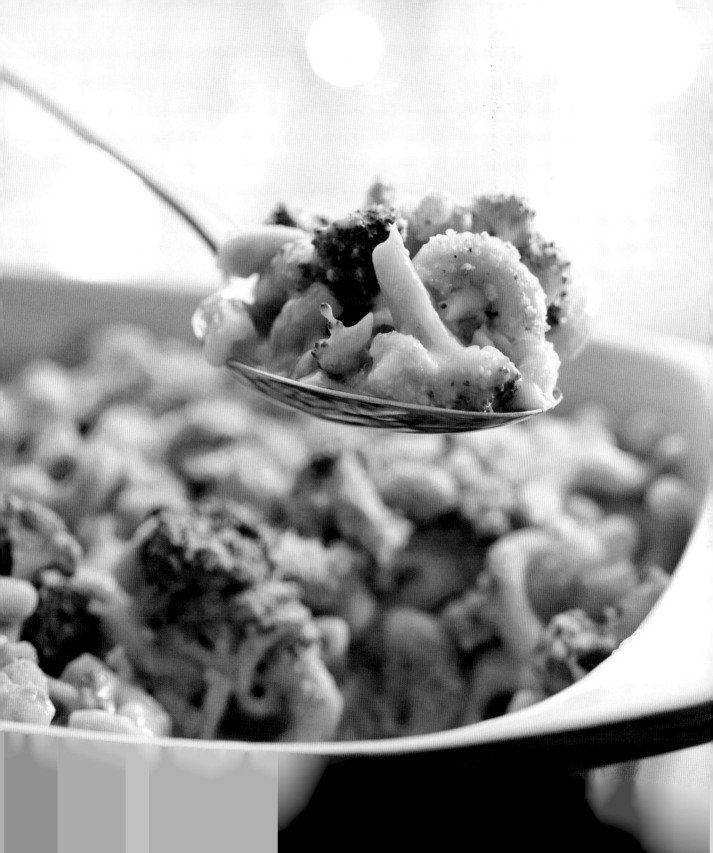

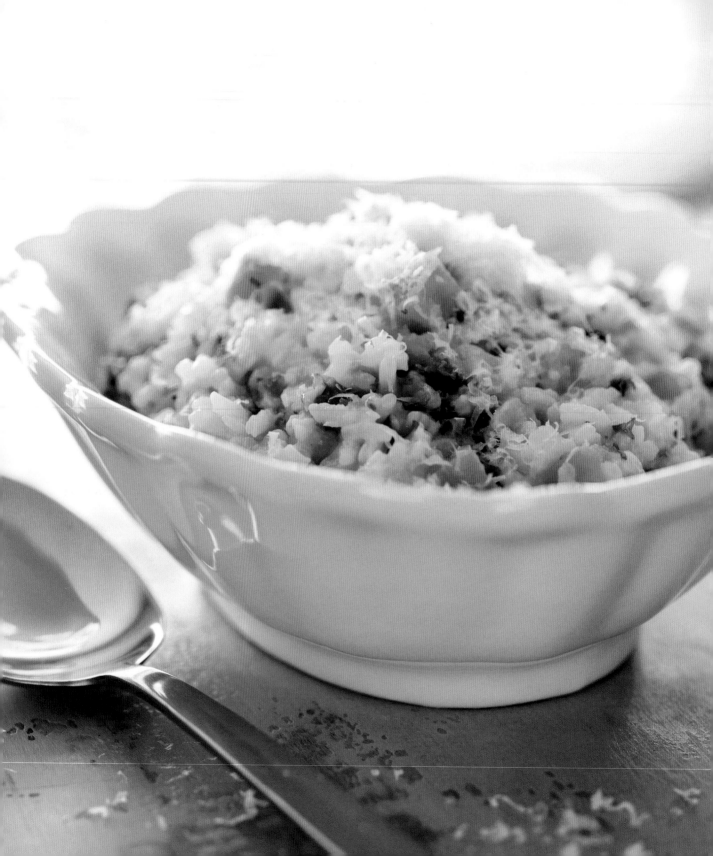

ITALIAN RICE Is Nice

RISOTTO WITH MUSHROOMS, BUTTERNUT SQUASH AND KALE

Risotto is my kind of comfort food. It's rich and filling, and the creamy texture soothes my soul. It's also a family favorite that everyone eats up, no matter how I make it. While most people associate risotto with expensive restaurants, the basic version of the dish is quite simple to make. If you can stir like mad, you can prepare a delicious risotto. The only catch is that it requires a little extra time, so I tend to make risotto on the weekends. When you see risotto on a menu, it may be part of the primi piatti, or first course, and sometimes you can order it as an entrée. This recipe has the flexibility to be enjoyed either way, especially since I've lightened up the traditional recipe that relies on liberal amounts of butter, stock, cheese and sometimes cream. By incorporating squash and kale, one serving provides 310 percent of your vitamin A needs, 100 percent of your vitamin C requirement and 30 percent of a day's worth of calcium.

YIELD: 4 servings | **TIME:** 1 hour

---

3 cups/450 g ½"/2.5 cm cubes butternut squash

2 tbsp/30 ml vegetable oil, divided

Salt and pepper

4 oz/112 g Tuscan kale, tough stems removed, roughly chopped

2 tbsp/28 g unsalted butter, divided

2 cups/160 g sliced cremini mushrooms

2 cups/320 g finely chopped onion

½ tsp rosemary, finely chopped

4 large cloves garlic, finely chopped

1 cup/190 g Arborio or Carnaroli rice

½ cup/120 ml white wine

4 cups/940 ml hot water

2 tsp/8 g lemon zest

1 tbsp/15 ml lemon juice

½ cup/50 g grated Parmigiano-Reggiano

Preheat oven to 400°F/200°C or gas mark 6. Place the butternut squash on a baking tray with 1 tablespoon/15 milliliters of the oil and a sprinkling of salt and pepper. Bake for about 20 minutes, turning the butternut squash once or twice, until a knife goes in easily and the cubes are golden. Set aside.

While the squash is cooking, place a medium pot of salted water over high heat and bring to a boil. Add the kale and simmer until tender, about 5 minutes. Drain the kale.

Heat a sauté pan over medium heat. Add 1 tablespoon/14 grams of the butter and a sprinkle of salt, and sauté the mushrooms until softened and beginning to brown, about 5 minutes.

Heat a large heavy-bottomed saucepan over medium heat. Add the remaining 1 tablespoon/14 grams butter and remaining 1 tablespoon/15 milliliters vegetable oil and sauté the onion until translucent, about 5 minutes. Add the rosemary and garlic and cook until aromatic, about 30 seconds. Stir in the Arborio rice and coat with the oil and butter. Increase heat to high and pour in the wine, stirring constantly. Sprinkle in ½ teaspoon salt. When most of the wine has been absorbed, stir in 1 ½ cups/350 milliliters of the water. Stir from time to time. When most of the water has been absorbed, add ½ cup/120 milliliters more water. Continue to add the water a little at a time. When ½ cup/120 milliliters water remains to be added, stir in the butternut squash, kale and mushrooms. Taste a few grains of rice and add more salt and pepper if needed and determine whether the rice is close to being cooked. It should be al dente when properly cooked. Add more water if needed. Just before serving, stir in lemon zest and juice and the cheese.

PER SERVING: Calories 430, protein 13 g, total fat 18 g, carbohydrates 59 g, sodium 280 mg, fiber 5 g

Tuscan **WINTER WARMER**

BEAN SOUP WITH KALE AND PARMESAN CHEESE RINDS

In my home, soup is comfort food that's always well received. Whether it's hearty and rustic or creamy and smooth, soup is heart-warming and nutritious. This recipe was inspired by the ingredients my family loves, which, when combined, makes a yummy stew that's a complete meal. My secret ingredient is the rind from a wedge of Parmesan cheese! Why toss the rind when you can use it for added flavor? Cheese rinds give soup added richness with few calories. For heartier, adult appetites, serve this soup with a nice green salad and glass of white wine. Of course, good bread is a must with soup. I like olive loaf, Asiago, multigrain or whole wheat dinner rolls.

YIELD: 12 servings | **TIME:** 2 hours 20 minutes

½ lb/230 g dried gigante beans or other dried white beans such as lima or cannellini

1 tbsp/15 ml olive oil

2 cups/320 g roughly chopped onion

2 oz/58 g finely chopped prosciutto

6 cloves garlic, finely chopped

1 tsp/1 g fresh rosemary, finely chopped

1 imported bay leaf

3oz/84 g Parmesan rind

1 ½ tsp/9 g salt

8 oz/224 g Tuscan kale or regular kale, roughly chopped

2 cups/360 g roughly chopped plum tomatoes

3 tbsp/12 g parsley, finely chopped

Grated cheese, for serving

Place beans in a large pot and cover with water by 2 inches/5 centimeters. Bring to a boil. Remove from heat and let stand, uncovered, for 1 hour. Drain beans in a colander, reserving some of the cooking liquid, and rinse.

Heat a soup pot over medium heat. Add the olive oil and sauté the onion until softened, about 5 minutes. Add the prosciutto, garlic and rosemary and cook, stirring, for another minute. Add the beans, water, bay leaf, cheese rind and salt, and simmer, uncovered, about 50 minutes, or until tender. Remove the bay leaf and discard. Take 1 cup/170 grams of the beans and cooking liquid and purée in a blender or food processor. Return to the pan.

Add the kale and tomatoes and continue to simmer, uncovered, stirring occasionally, until kale is soft, about 10 minutes. Taste soup and season, if needed, with salt and pepper. This soup only gets better as it continues to cook, so if there's time, simmer longer, adding more water as needed. Serve in soup bowls topped with parsley and generous amounts of grated cheese.

PER SERVING: Calories 100, protein 6 g, total fat 2 g, carbohydrates 16 g, sodium 140 mg, fiber 5 g

TINA'S TIP: Dried beans store well, so it's worth having a few varieties on hand to hydrate and add to soup or chili. For added flavor, you can sauté the kale first in olive oil before adding it to the soup.

GET FIGGIE WITH IT

FIG, ARUGULA AND BRIE FLATBREAD

On those rare occasions when I have the house to myself and I can enjoy the company of my girlfriends, I like to make something that's easy; I certainly don't want to spend what little free time I have in the kitchen. I also want to make something healthy. It's what everyone expects, and they look forward to trying something new that they can add to their own recipe file. This recipe is like a gourmet salad atop a pizza crust. It's waistline-friendly, yet the Brie and figs give it a special, "girl's night" touch. Served with a nice white wine, this pizza is a lovely, low-stress meal that pleases every palate!

YIELD: 8 servings | **TIME:** 30 minutes

1 ½ tsp/7.5 ml olive oil

5 oz/140 g arugula

¼ tsp salt

Flour, as needed

1 lb/455 g pizza dough, at room temperature

3 oz/85 g Brie, cut into small pieces

12 fresh figs

1½ tsp/7.5 ml balsamic vinegar

Preheat oven to 450°F/230°C or gas mark 8.

In a large sauté pan, warm olive oil over medium-high heat. Add half the arugula, sautéing for about 1 minute to wilt. Add remaining arugula and salt, continuing to sauté to wilt. Remove from heat and reserve.

Layer a rimmed 12 x 16-inch/30 x 40-centimeter baking sheet with foil and coat with cooking spray. Sprinkle 1 to 2 tablespoons/8 to 16 grams of flour onto a cutting board, and dust both sides of pizza dough with flour. Slowly stretch the dough on the back of your knuckles, rotating the dough and stretching it out into a rectangular shape to fit the baking sheet. When the dough is stretched out to about 12 inches/30 centimeters, place on the baking sheet and stretch the pizza dough further using your fingertips.

Dot with Brie pieces. Next, spread the entire flatbread with reserved arugula. Trim the stem from each fig, and cut into 3 slices. Place fig slices over arugula. Bake until flatbread is golden brown, about 12 to 15 minutes. Remove from oven, drizzle with vinegar and let cool. Cut into 8 pieces, and serve.

PER SERVING: Calories 240, protein 7 g, total fat 6 g, carbohydrates 43 g, sodium 330 mg, fiber 4 g

TINA'S TIP: While I enjoy the peppery "bite" of arugula, spinach can be substituted, if you prefer.

SEE FOOD Your Way

MOCK BOUILLABAISSE THREE WAYS

The classic bouillabaisse recipe is typically long and involved, but my shortcut version saves time without sacrificing taste. Normally, bouillabaisse uses a minimum of five different types of fish, and a mixture of finfish and shellfish, but my version uses just four types of shellfish, all of which can be found at your local grocer year-round. I suggest buying "dry-packed" scallops because commonly, scallops are soaked in a phosphate solution that brightens their color and makes them absorb more liquid (so you pay more). It also changes their natural taste profile, so ask for dry-packed or chemical-free scallops. Armed with plastic bibs and fish forks, kids of all ages will enjoy this fun to eat and richly satisfying stew that delivers protein, nutrients and essential fats to the diet.

YIELD: 4 servings   **TIME:** 30 minutes

2 tsp/10 ml olive oil

¼ cup/40 g finely chopped shallot

2 tsp/6 g finely chopped garlic

½ tsp thyme leaves

¼ tsp saffron strands

1 cup/240 ml white wine

4 cups/940 ml fish stock

2 cups/360 g roughly chopped tomatoes

12 clams

12 mussels

8 "dry/chemical-free" sea scallops, halved

8 medium shrimp

¼ cup/15 g parsley, chopped

Heat a large soup pot over medium-high heat. Add the olive oil and sauté the shallot until softened and starting to brown, about 3 minutes. Add the garlic, thyme and saffron and continue to cook until aromatic, about 30 seconds. Deglaze the pan with the wine. Cook until reduced by half, about 10 minutes. Add fish stock and tomatoes. Bring to a boil, then reduce to a simmer and cook another 5 minutes, allowing the flavors to meld. Add the clams. Cook until most have opened and then add the mussels. When most of the mussels have opened, add the scallops and shrimp. Cook for another 2 minutes. The shrimp should be pink. Discard any clams or mussels that fail to open. Add the parsley and serve.

THREE SERVING OPTIONS:

• This is delicious with a green salad and crusty bread.

• Serve over rice or couscous (½ cup/80 grams per person).

• To make the stew thicker with more body, stir in ¼ cup/30 grams plain breadcrumbs with the mussels.

PER SERVING: Calories 390, protein 43 g, total fat 12 g, carbohydrates 12 g, sodium 740 mg, fiber 1 g

TINA'S TIP: Canned tomatoes (15 ounces/420 grams) can be substituted for fresh tomatoes. They will give a substantially more tomato-y flavor, which is equally delicious but just a little different.

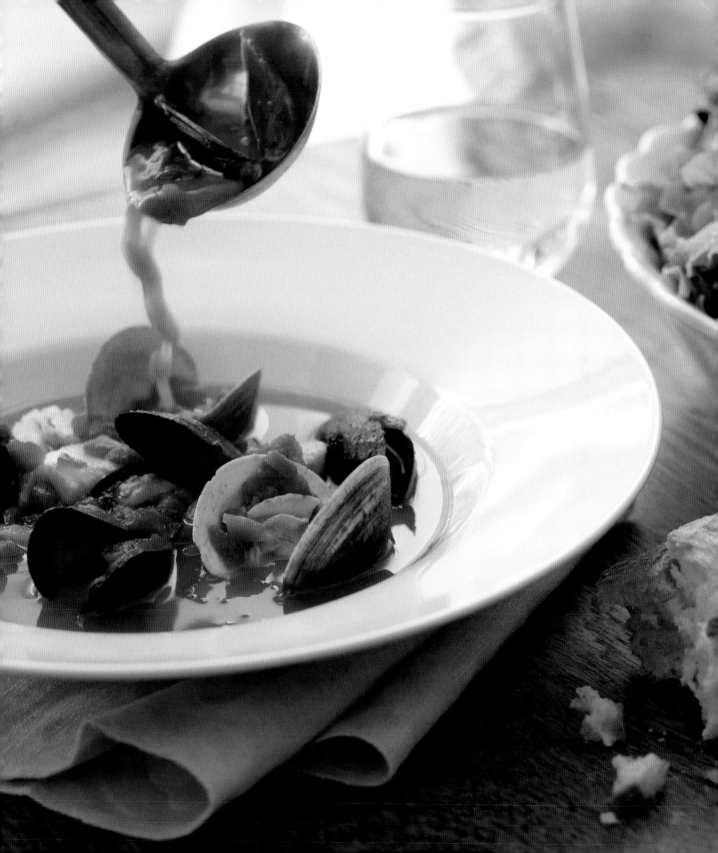

SPANISH Eyes

ARROZ CON POLLO WITH GREEN CHILES AND PINTO BEANS

This traditional Latin American dish has become a classic in my home, because it's always guaranteed to please. I've adapted it slightly, making a delicious sauce with the veggies and using skinless chicken and brown rice to deliver more nutrients and less fat. Thanks to the tender, slow-cooked chicken, beans and herbs, this dish will surely get you a gold star! The fact that it's a one-pot meal makes it even more appealing. Active cooking time is minimal, and cleanup is quick. Each portion delivers important nutrients in a small serving, along with 25 percent of your daily iron needs, 15 percent of your calcium requirements and almost half of your daily vitamin C needs.

YIELD: 4 servings | **TIME:** 1 hour 15 minutes

1 medium onion, roughly chopped

2 cloves garlic, peeled

2 (5 oz/140 g) cans diced or whole mild green chiles

1 cup/16 g cilantro, roughly chopped and packed

¼ cup/60 ml lime juice

½ tsp salt, plus more for sprinkling

¼ cup/60 ml water

4 (4 oz/112 g) skinless, bone-in chicken thighs

Freshly ground pepper

1 ½ cups/355 ml low-sodium chicken broth or water

1 cup/190 g brown rice

1 (15.5 oz/434 g) can pinto beans, rinsed and drained

Place onion, garlic, chiles, cilantro, lime juice, salt and water in a blender or food processor and purée until smooth. Reserve.

Sprinkle the chicken thighs with a little salt and pepper on both sides. Place the reserved green sauce, broth, rice and chicken thighs in a medium-size soup pot. Bring to a simmer, cover and cook for 30 minutes. Check to make sure the pan isn't drying out. Stir in the beans and continue to cook for another 10 to 15 minutes, or until the rice is cooked. Divide among 4 bowls.

PER SERVING: Calories 410, protein 29 g, total fat 6 g, carbohydrates 54 g, sodium 810 mg, fiber 7 g

TINA'S TIP: For a sweeter, slightly smoky variation of this recipe, try substituting roasted red peppers and 2 teaspoons of chipotle puree for the green chilies. And if you've made this recipe for adults, pair it with a nice Sancerre or Pinot Noir for red wine lovers.

Keep Your Eye on
THE PIZZA PIE

GORGONZOLA AND SWEET ONION PIZZA WITH ARUGULA AND BALSAMIC STRAWBERRIES

Pizza is usually considered junk food, but that's not the case in my house. Homemade pizza is far more nutritious than what you might find in your supermarket freezer or fast food restaurant. Loaded with veggies and even fruit, pizza can provide significant nutrition in a very small portion. In just one slice of this savory flatbread, you get nearly 25 percent of a day's calcium requirement and 15 percent of your iron needs. It's also a good source of protein, and the mixture of flavors and textures makes it very satisfying. To save time, you can purchase freshly prepared dough from your local pizza parlor.

YIELD: 1 (12"/30 cm) pie, 6 servings | **TIME:** 45 minutes

4 oz/112 g Gorgonzola, at room temperature

6 oz/170 g part-skim ricotta, at room temperature

½ tsp rosemary, finely chopped

Freshly ground black pepper

Cornmeal for sprinkling

1 lb/455 g prepared pizza dough

½ medium yellow onion, sliced very thinly into rounds

¼ cup/60 ml balsamic vinegar

2 cups/40 g arugula

1 ¼ cups/213 g sliced strawberries

Preheat oven to 500°F/250°C or gas mark 10. Place the Gorgonzola, ricotta and rosemary in a bowl along with several grinds of black pepper, and mix to thoroughly combine. Sprinkle a 12-inch/30-centimeter round baking tray (or other baking tray that will fit a 12-inch/30-centimeter circle of dough) with a little cornmeal. Stretch the pizza dough into a 12-inch/30-centimeter circle, leaving the edge a little thicker. Spread the cheese mixture over the dough, leaving a 1-inch/2.5-centimeter border. Top with the onions and place in the oven. Bake until the crust is golden and cooked through and the cheese is bubbling and browning in spots, about 20 minutes.

While the pizza is baking, pour balsamic vinegar into a small saucepan. Simmer until it is reduced by half. It should be syrupy and sweet.

Allow the pizza to cool and set for 5 to 10 minutes before topping with arugula, strawberries and 2 teaspoons/10 milliliters of the balsamic glaze.

PER SERVING: Calories 290, protein 13 g, total fat 11 g, carbohydrates 40 g, sodium 550 mg, fiber 2 g

TINA'S TIP: Keep the extra balsamic glaze that you don't use in this recipe. It's delicious drizzled over fruit such as fresh figs and peaches, or rich fish like salmon and sea bass.

RAT-A-TAT-TAT

RATATOUILLE AND BULGUR-STUFFED EGGPLANT

When I was growing up, eggplant was practically a staple, like butter, milk and eggs. My grandmother was always preparing the versatile veggie, stuffing, baking, frying, grilling or chopping it for soup or caponata. Needless to say, this book would not be complete without an eggplant recipe! This one reflects the preferred flavors in my home, and I'm certain these "eggplant boats" will become a favorite meal in your household, too. Of course, the dish is very healthy. The antioxidant nasunin, which gives the eggplant its glorious color, is a powerful, cancer-fighting compound. Bulgur, a whole grain, delivers a nutty flavor and a hearty, chewy texture, and combined with all of the other ingredients, you have a flavorful, fiber-rich meal that will satisfy even the biggest of appetites.

YIELD: 4 servings | **TIME:** 1 hour 15 minutes

2 small to medium eggplants

½ cup/80 g bulgur

1 cup/235 ml boiling water

1 tbsp/15 ml extra-virgin olive oil

2 cups/320 g roughly chopped onion

Salt and freshly ground pepper

¼ cup/40 g roughly chopped garlic

2 tsp/2 g thyme leaves

2 cups/240 g diced zucchini

2 cups/240 g diced yellow squash

4 cups/720 g roughly chopped tomato

6 tbsp/15 g basil, sliced and divided

¼ cup/25 g grated Parmigiano-Reggiano

Cut eggplants in half lengthwise. Using the tip of a knife, cut out the flesh of the eggplant, leaving a ¼-inch/6-millimeter border to hold the eggplant intact. Angle the blade to help avoid poking through the skin. Use a spoon to scrape out any additional flesh and seeds. Roughly chop the eggplant flesh. Place the eggplants on a baking sheet and set aside.

Place bulgur in a bowl and cover with the boiling water. Cover bowl. Let stand for at least 15 minutes.

Preheat oven to 350°F/180°C or gas mark 4. Heat a large sauté pan over medium heat. Add the olive oil and sauté the onion, sprinkling with some salt and pepper, until lightly browned, about 3 minutes. Add the garlic and thyme, and cook until aromatic, 1 minute more. Add the eggplant, sprinkle with additional salt, lower heat, cover and cook until softened, stirring once or twice, about 8 minutes. Increase heat to medium and add the zucchini and yellow squash and a sprinkle of salt. Cook, stirring occasionally, until they start to brown, about 5 minutes. Stir in tomatoes and 4 tablespoons/10 grams of the basil. Bring to a simmer and cook for 10 minutes. Stir the bulgur into the ratatouille. Divide among the eggplants. Sprinkle with cheese and remaining 2 tablespoons/5 grams basil. Bake for 40 minutes, or until the eggplant is soft and the filling is heated through.

PER SERVING: Calories 200, protein 8 g, total fat 6 g, carbohydrates 30 g, sodium 170 mg, fiber 7 g

TINA'S TIP: Ratatouille can also make a lovely appetizer baked in a tart shell.

BUNDLES OF *Joy*

SWISS CHARD BUNDLES STUFFED WITH GROUND TURKEY AND COUSCOUS

This dark green vegetable with rainbow-colored stalks delivers plenty of nutrients per bite—from vitamins A, C and K to fiber and disease-fighting phytochemicals. Tender enough to enjoy raw in a salad, cooked, it's the perfect foil for just about any ingredient! Here I use Swiss chard to wrap up tasty morsels of ground turkey, fluffy couscous and savory feta cheese. Each portion provides 70 percent vitamin A, 30 percent vitamin C and 10 percent iron.

YIELD: 12 bundles, 6 servings | **TIME:** 45 minutes

½ cup/88 g uncooked whole wheat couscous

2 bunches Swiss chard, stems trimmed* and washed

½ tbsp/7.5 ml olive oil

1 lb/455 g ground turkey

1 tsp/2.2 g ground turmeric

¾ tsp ground cumin

½ tsp kosher salt

⅓ cup/100 g golden raisins

⅓ cup/50 g plus 1½ tbsp/14 g crumbled feta cheese, divided

1 cup/160 g crushed tomatoes

Fill a large pot with water, and bring to a boil over high heat. Add couscous to a small bowl, and carefully ladle ¾ cup/180 milliliters hot water into couscous. Tightly cover with plastic wrap or foil, and let sit 10 minutes. Then, using tongs, add Swiss chard leaves to boiling water in 2 or 3 batches, cooking each batch just 1 minute to wilt. Transfer each batch of leaves into a bowl of cold water to shock leaves.

Preheat oven to 400°F/200°C or gas mark 6. In a medium sauté pan, warm oil over medium-high heat. Add turkey, turmeric, cumin and salt. Stir to combine and break turkey up into small pieces until fully cooked, about 7 minutes. Remove ground turkey from heat, and transfer to a medium bowl. Stir in raisins, ⅓ cup/50 grams feta cheese and reserved couscous.

To prepare Swiss chard bundles, drain Swiss chard leaves from water, patting them with paper towels to remove a bit of water. Lay 1 Swiss chard leaf on a cutting board horizontally. Spoon a few tablespoons (about 42 grams) of mixture in a vertical strip onto one side of the leaf. As tightly as you can, roll the bottom of the leaf up over filling, tucking it in. Then, fold over each side, the top first, and then the bottom. Continue rolling the leaf until entire piece is rolled into a small bundle. Transfer to a baking dish. Continue until all of the filling is used (not all the Swiss chard may be used). Sprinkle remaining 1½ tablespoons/14 grams feta cheese over bundles, and top with crushed tomatoes. Bake for 20 minutes, or until heated through, and serve.

* Save the stems to sauté in a stir-fry.

PER BUNDLE: Calories 120, protein 13 g, total fat 2 g, carbohydrates 13 g, sodium 360 mg, fiber 3 g

TINA'S TIP: Save any broken or small Swiss chard leaves to incorporate into a smoothie or toss into a salad.

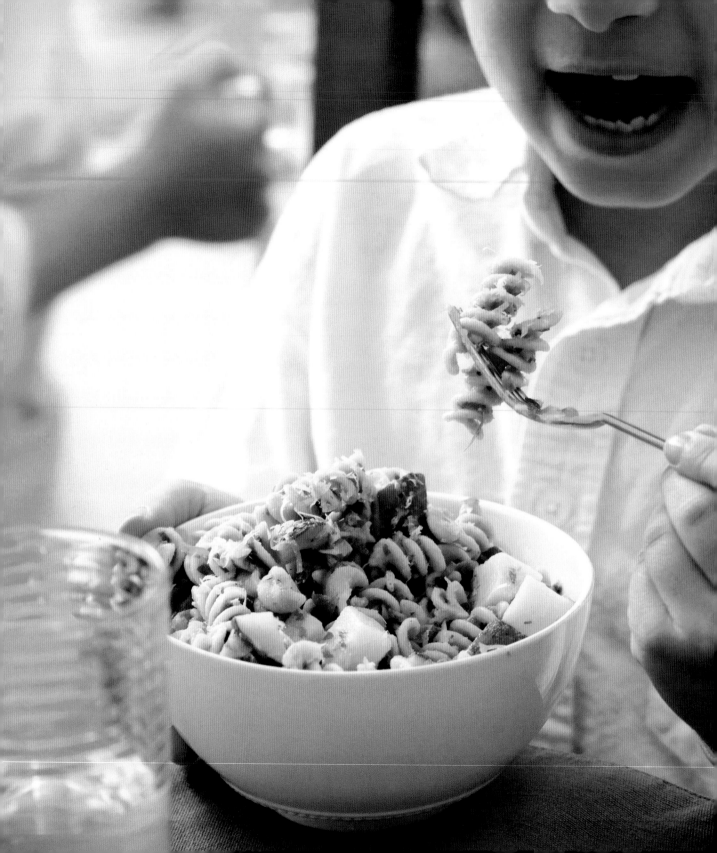

Silly **FUSILLI**

PASTA WITH GREEN BEANS, POTATOES AND GREMOLATA

I like dishes that can be served hot or cold. It makes things easier for me when I know I have something in the refrigerator that can be quickly heated for dinner or put into a container as part of a healthy, brown bag lunch. This is one of those recipes that does double duty, and it can last several days in the refrigerator—another perk! This recipe is inspired by gremolata, a condiment of Italian origin, which includes garlic, lemon juice and parsley. Those ingredients, whirled in a food processor, make the sauce for this dish. Combined with red potatoes, green beans and fusilli, you have an unforgettable meal! And if you've never had potatoes with pasta, you're in for a treat. The ingredients are perfect together, and they make a very nutritious meal, which satisfies 35 percent of your daily vitamin C needs and 20 percent of your vitamin A requirement.

YIELD: 4 servings | **TIME:** 40 minutes

1 lb/455 g red potatoes, diced into 1"/2.5 cm cubes

3½ tbsp/52.5 ml olive oil, divided

Salt and freshly ground pepper

1 clove garlic, roughly chopped

1½ cups/90 g parsley leaves

2 tbsp/12 g lemon zest

1 tbsp/15 ml lemon juice

10 oz/280 g whole wheat fusilli or other small pasta

2 cups/200 g chopped green beans

Parmigiano-Reggiano, finely grated, for serving

Preheat oven to 425°F/220°C or gas mark 7. On a baking sheet, place potato cubes and drizzle with ½ tablespoon/7.5 milliliters of the oil, and season with salt and pepper. Roast potatoes in oven until cooked but still meet slight resistance when pierced with a knife, about 15 minutes, stirring the potatoes at the halfway mark. Remove from oven and reserve.

Meanwhile, to make gremolata, add garlic and parsley to the bowl of a food processor. Pulse until the parsley is finely chopped, about 30 seconds. Add lemon zest and lemon juice. Purée mixture, pouring the remaining 3 tablespoons/45 milliliters olive oil through the feeder tube. Stop food processor, scrape mixture down with spatula, and purée again. Reserve.

Bring a large pot of salted water to a boil over high heat. Add pasta, and cook for 7 minutes. Add green beans into the pot with pasta, cooking until the pasta is al dente, about 3 more minutes. Reserve ¼ cup/60 milliliters of pasta water. Then, drain pasta and green beans in colander. Return pasta and green beans to the pot. Stir in reserved potatoes, gremolata, and reserved pasta water, combining until gremolata coats the pasta. Season with salt and pepper to taste. Top generously with cheese, and serve.

PER SERVING: Calories 150, protein 4 g, total fat 6 g, carbohydrates 21 g, sodium 15 mg, fiber 3 g

TINA'S TIP: Orecchiette is another pasta shape that works very well with this type of sauce.

MEATLESS Madness

BLACK BEAN BURGER WITH CHIPOTLE AND CILANTRO

Today, many people are trying to incorporate more plant-based foods into their diet, and beans are an ideal ingredient. Beans are very similar to meat, poultry and fish in terms of their iron and zinc content; they're an excellent source of fiber, folate and potassium, and they make sense for your wallet. My family just thinks they taste great! On "Meatless Mondays," we enjoy these bean burgers, which everyone customizes to his or her own taste. I like mine open-face with sliced avocado and Greek yogurt; my husband likes his with hot peppers and low-fat sour cream; and the kids opt for romaine, fresh tomato and Cheddar cheese. Whichever way you enjoy this recipe, it provides mega nutrition and satisfaction!

YIELD: 6 burgers   **TIME:** 30 minutes

¼ cup/56 g nonfat Greek yogurt

2 tsp/5 g ground cumin

2 tsp/10 ml chipotle purée, or more to taste (optional)

2 (15 oz/420 g) cans black beans, rinsed and drained, divided

¾ cup/86 g plain dry breadcrumbs, divided

½ cup/8 g cilantro, leaves and stems, finely chopped

Salt and freshly ground pepper

1 tbsp/15 ml vegetable oil

6 whole wheat hamburger buns

Place the yogurt, cumin, chipotle, three-fourths of the beans and ⅓ cup/ 38 grams of the breadcrumbs in a food processor and pulse until a coarse purée forms. Transfer to a bowl and stir in cilantro and remaining one-fourth beans. Taste bean mixture and season to taste with salt, pepper and more chipotle purée, if desired. Form mixture into 6 patties, adding more of the remaining breadcrumbs if necessary. Mixture should be fairly dry, not sticky. Pat breadcrumbs onto the outside of each bean burger patty.

Heat a large sauté pan over medium heat. Add vegetable oil to coat the bottom of the pan. Cook bean burgers until outsides are crisp and lightly browned, about 2 minutes per side. Toast the burger buns, place the burgers in the buns and garnish as desired.

PER BURGER: Calories 190, protein 11 g, total fat 3 g, carbohydrates 30 g, sodium 130 mg, fiber 7 g

TINA'S TIP: Try making these burgers with brown lentils. Overcook them slightly, so they will break down easily in the food processor. A mixture of black beans and lentils is a nice option, as well.

The Marvelous
MEDITERRANEAN

BAKED FETTUCCINE WITH SHRIMP, ARTICHOKE, BROCCOLI RABE, TOMATO AND RICOTTA

I rarely, if ever, order baked pasta when I go out to eat. The dish tends to be very high in fat and sodium, drowning in cheese and filled with greasy meat. I prefer to make homemade baked pasta that's brimming with nutrients, lots of flavor and simple ingredients I know everyone loves. It's lovely for a luncheon yet suitable for Easter; it will impress the in-laws, and I've served it as a "welcome back" dinner for hungry collegiates happy to enjoy home cooking once again. By incorporating broccoli rabe, also called rapini or broccoletti, this dish takes on a slightly nutty flavor and good amounts of vitamins A and K, 100% of a day's worth of vitamin C and the minerals potassium, calcium and iron. Tomatoes contribute lycopene, artichokes add vital antioxidants and shrimp contributes lean protein. The result? A smart comfort food for the body and soul.

YIELD: 8 servings | **TIME:** 50 minutes

1 tbsp/15 ml extra-virgin olive oil

2 cups/320 g medium dice onion

2 cloves garlic, finely chopped

1 tsp thyme leaves

½ tsp red pepper flakes

2 tbsp/32 g tomato paste

½ cup/120 ml white wine

1 (28 oz/784 g) can plum tomatoes

3 cups/210 g roughly chopped broccoli rabe (tough stems removed)

1 lb/454 g fettuccine

2 cups/600 g jarred artichokes, quartered

1 (15 oz/420 g) tub part-skim ricotta

32 medium shrimp

1 cup/100 g grated Parmigiano-Reggiano

Preheat the oven to 400°F/200°C or gas mark 6. Bring a large pot of salted water to a boil over medium-high heat. While it's heating, start the tomato sauce. Heat a saucepan over medium heat, add the oil and sauté the onion until softened and beginning to brown, about 5 minutes. Add the garlic, thyme and pepper flakes, and cook until aromatic, about 30 seconds. Add the tomato paste and stir to caramelize slightly. Add the wine and tomatoes, breaking them up. Bring to a simmer and cook until thickened slightly, about 10 minutes.

Add the broccoli rabe to the boiling water and cook until softened, 3 minutes. Strain out the broccoli rabe but save the water to cook the pasta. Reserve.

Cook the pasta following the manufacturer's recommendation but cook it 1 minute less than recommended for al dente.

To build the baked fettuccine, place half the fettuccine along the bottom of a 9 x 13-inch/23 x 33-centimeter pan. Ladle half the tomato sauce over the pasta. Strew half the broccoli rabe and half the artichokes over the sauce. Spoon half the ricotta in 8 evenly spaced spoonfuls over the vegetables. Place 2 shrimp on top of each ricotta. Repeat. Finish by sprinkling with the Parmigiano-Reggiano. Bake for 20 minutes, or until the shrimp are cooked through and everything is nice and hot. Allow to cool slightly before serving.

PER BURGER: Calories 510, protein 33 g, total fat 13 g, carbohydrates 58 g, sodium 760 mg, fiber 4 g

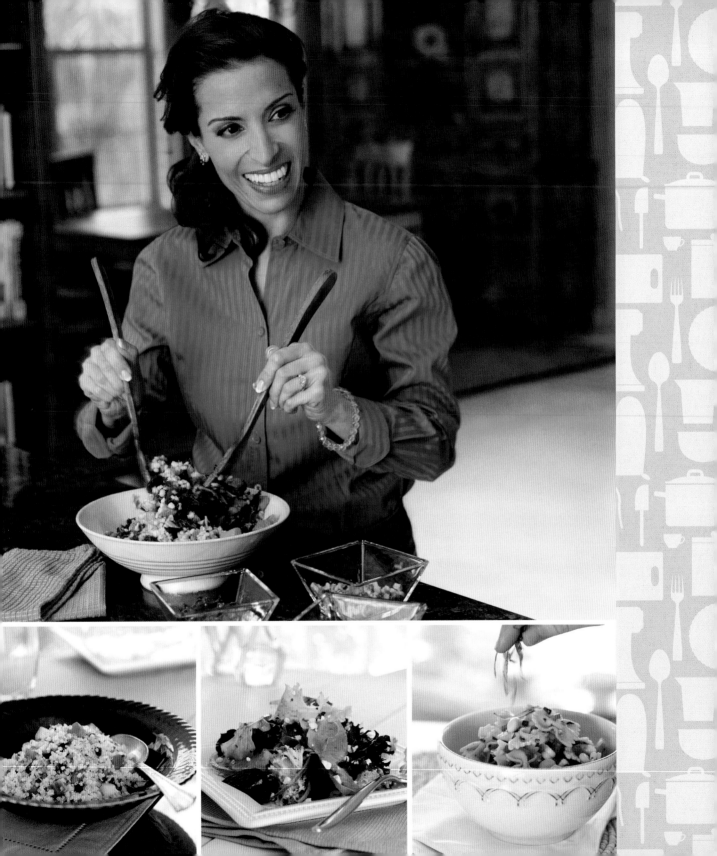

Simply Sensational Salad Meals and Side Dishes

Give mealtime a makeover with exciting recipes that deliver health and deliciousness!

Side dishes can be transformative. They can make a simple meal sensational. They can make an old favorite seem new. They can add color, nutrition and flavor to a humble supper. In my opinion, sides dishes are unsung heroes, and they're sometimes more satisfying than the main attraction!

When I develop a side dish—or any recipe, for that matter—I'm not interested in creating one that's "low-fat," "low-calorie," or "free" from this or that; these criteria don't necessarily mean the meal will be healthy. I consider taste first, but then I think about nutrition, asking myself: Will the dish contribute essential vitamins and minerals to my diet? Is it rich in heart-healthy fats? Will it fight disease or boost immunity? How will it benefit my family? Then, I get busy in the kitchen ...

To pack the most taste and nutrition into every little bite of the sides and salads you'll find on the following pages, I played with new ingredients or tried different things with familiar sides, giving them a bit of a makeover. The results are incredible, and I promise they'll please even the pickiest of eaters. If there are any ingredients in my recipes you haven't heard of or tried before, give them a go! Odds are, you'll discover a new taste sensation that will also incorporate more health and satisfaction into your family meals.

If you crave sides and salads that are fresh and different, hassle-free and healthy, the pages of this chapter are filled with what you're looking for.

Wild ABOUT VEGGIES

WILD MUSHROOMS AND ASPARAGUS WITH SESAME SEEDS

I love the humble, little mushroom. Its role in health is growing every day, as new science suggests this vegetable may protect us from certain cancers. In this recipe, crisp asparagus is the perfect complement to tender mushrooms, and the asparagus also contributes vitamins D and K, vitamins that actually need one another to act efficiently in the body. A sprinkle of sesame seeds adds fiber and crunch, and you have a truly healthy, satisfying side to pair with fish, chicken or shrimp!

YIELD: 4 servings   **TIME:** 15 minutes

2 tsp/10 ml vegetable oil

¼ cup/40 g thinly sliced onion

Salt

2 cups/200 g mixed wild mushrooms, sliced in ¼"/6 mm lengths

4 cloves garlic, thinly sliced

2 cups/240 g asparagus, diagonally sliced in 1 ½"/3.8 cm lengths

2 tbsp/30 ml mirin or white wine

2 tsp/10 ml soy sauce

1 ½ tsp/4 g toasted sesame seeds (black and white are particularly dramatic)

2 tsp/10 ml sesame oil

Heat a sauté pan over medium heat. Add the vegetable oil and the onion. Sprinkle with a little salt. Allow to soften and brown slightly, about 1 minute. Add the mushrooms and a sprinkle of salt and continue to cook, shaking the pan to turn the mushrooms. Allow the mushrooms to soften and brown slightly, about 2 minutes. Add the garlic and asparagus and continue to cook another 30 seconds. Deglaze the pan with the mirin and soy sauce. Toss in the sesame seeds and sesame oil. Cook for another minute, or until the asparagus is crisp and tender.

PER SERVING: Calories 80, protein 3 g, total fat 5 g, carbohydrates 6 g, sodium 80 mg, fiber 2 g

TINA'S TIP: Riesling is a great wine with a flowery aroma, and is a lovely accompaniment to this dish.

Can't **BEET THIS!**

BEETS AND THEIR GREENS WITH LEMON AND ALMONDS

It never fails. When friends come to my home for lunch and bring their children, they'll often laugh at what I'm cooking and jokingly say, "Tina, if my kids eat that, I'll pay you!" Nine times out of ten, the kids gobble up what I've made. This is one of those "I can't believe they ate it" side dishes. Sautéed beet greens are delicious when cooked properly; the leafy tops and stems can stretch your budget, and they add a ton of nutrients to meals. Just 1 cup/70 grams of beet greens provides more than 25 percent of your daily requirement for potassium, magnesium and vitamin A. And, they add gorgeous color to your plate.

YIELD: 4 servings | **TIME:** 40 minutes

1 bunch beets with greens

1 tbsp/15 ml extra-virgin olive oil

1 clove garlic, finely chopped

½ tsp thyme leaves

2 tbsp/14 g finely chopped toasted almonds

1 tbsp/15 ml lemon juice

1 tbsp/4 g parsley, roughly chopped

Salt

Cut the beet greens away from the beets. Slice them into 1-inch/2.5-centimeter strips and rinse well. Place in a pot of salted water, bring to a boil and cook until the beets are soft, about 30 minutes, depending on the size of the beets. Remove the beets from the water. Place the beet greens in the boiling water and cook until softened, about 5 minutes. Drain. Peel the beets and cut into bite-size pieces.

Heat a sauté pan over medium heat. Add the olive oil, garlic and thyme. As soon as the garlic begins to sizzle, add the beet greens and then the beets. Toss to slightly crisp up the beets and the greens. Add the almonds, drizzle with lemon juice and sprinkle wih parsley. Season with salt to taste.

PER SERVING: Calories 120, protein 3 g, total fat 5 g, carbohydrates 18 g, sodium 315 mg, fiber 5 g

TINA'S TIP: To avoid purple fingers, use gloves when peeling the beets. Just rub the skins, and they will slip right off! And if you prefer to roast the beets, that will work, too. I like to boil the beets in this recipe, then use the water for homemade vegetable stock. Delicious!

Savory SEA VEGGIE SALAD

ASIAN-INSPIRED WAKAME SALAD

Asian cultures have been enjoying sea vegetables for centuries. In the Western world, we're just getting to know and appreciate these marine veggies for their taste and health-boosting powers. You can find a basic assortment of sea vegetables online or in your local health food store. There's nori, used in sushi; kelp, frequently found in flake or powdered form; hijiki, which looks like strands of black angel hair pasta; lacy arame; soft and chewy dulse; and wakame, which is used in miso soup. Each type of sea vegetable acts as an antioxidant. They also may play a role in cancer prevention and appear to have the ability to stabilize blood pressure. Those facts, combined with their rich mineral content, make them a smart addition to your diet!

YIELD: 4 servings | **TIME:** 30 minutes

1 oz/28 g wakame

3 tbsp/45 ml unseasoned rice vinegar

2 tsp/10 ml sesame oil

1 tsp/3 g grated ginger

1 tsp/4 g sugar

½ tsp salt

2 cups/160 g mesclun

1 cup/120 g diced cucumber

½ cup/55 g julienned or grated carrot

½ cup/50 g thinly sliced scallion

½ cup/75 g diced avocado

Place the wakame in a medium bowl and cover with plenty of hot tap water. Wakame will expand quite a bit. Let sit for 15 minutes, or until softened. Drain and roughly chop into bite-size pieces.

While wakame is rehydrating, make the vinaigrette. Whisk together the rice vinegar, sesame oil, ginger, sugar and salt. Set aside.

Place wakame, mesclun, cucumber, carrot, scallion and avocado in a bowl. Toss with vinaigrette. Divide among 4 salad plates.

PER SERVING: Calories 80, protein 3 g, total fat 5 g, carbohydrates 8 g, sodium 480 mg, fiber 5 g

TINA'S TIP: Seaweed isn't just for salad; it is a delicious addition to soups and stir-fries.

Rosie's **BETTER BEANS**

BUTTER BEANS WITH TOMATOES, GARLIC, ROSEMARY AND OLIVE OIL

Busy weeknights call for quick meals, and this recipe is perfect because it cooks while I'm sorting mail, doing laundry or writing another one of my "to do" lists. When it's time for dinner, the entire family will clamor for this sensational side, which goes well with everything from roast chicken and fish to pork chops and juicy hamburgers. And you don't have to feel guilty about having seconds! Low in fat, high in fiber and rich in minerals, this combination of simple ingredients delivers heaps of health!

YIELD: 6 servings | **TIME:** 1 hour

8 oz/224 g dried butter beans (also called gigante beans or large lima beans)

10 cloves garlic, smashed

2 sprigs rosemary

2 cups/320 g roughly chopped tomatoes

½ tsp salt

2 tbsp/30 ml extra-virgin olive oil

1 cup/235 ml water

Place beans in a large saucepan. Cover with cold water and bring to a boil. Remove from heat and let sit for 30 minutes. Drain the beans. Place them back in the pan with the garlic, rosemary, tomatoes, salt, olive oil and the water. Bring to a simmer and cover. Cook until beans are soft, about 30 minutes, stirring once or twice. Taste and adjust seasoning. Remove rosemary before serving.

PER SERVING: Calories 100, protein 4 g, total fat 5 g, carbohydrates 12 g, sodium 200 mg, fiber 3 g

TINA'S TIP: To make a delicious white bean dip, cook the beans until softened and breaking apart, then purée them in a food processor until smooth, along with the remaining ingredients in this recipe. Serve with toasted bread and veggies.

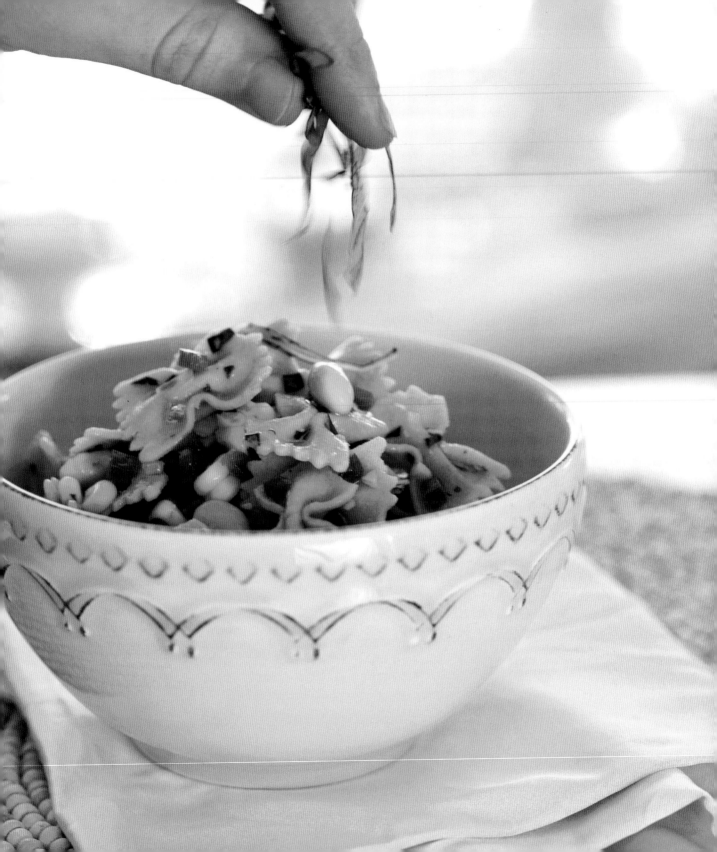

Confetti **FARFALLE**

WHOLE WHEAT PASTA WITH EDAMAME, CORN, RED PEPPER AND BASIL

Pasta is a great source of carbohydrates, the brain's and body's most vital energy source. Plus, pasta is a favorite among kids. Just be sure to cook it *al dente*; nothing is more unappealing than soggy pasta, especially when it's in pasta salad. While most recipes for this dish are uninspired, having too much mayo or vinegar, my recipe is very different. Crunchy vegetables give this salad a satisfying texture; the marinade is light and delicate; fresh basil provides a wonderful aroma; and edamame—the only veggie that contains all nine essential amino acids—adds a good dose of vitamins A and C and the minerals calcium and iron. If you don't have farfalle, feel free to just use another small pasta. No matter how you prepare it, this dish will be a colorful and happy addition to any table.

YIELD: 4 servings | **TIME:** 30 minutes

⅓ cup/53 g finely chopped shallots

2 tsp/8 g grainy Dijon mustard

1 tbsp/15 ml red wine vinegar

3 tbsp/45 ml extra-virgin olive oil

2 ears corn or 1 cup/130 g fresh corn kernels

4 oz/112 g whole wheat farfalle, cooked according to package directions

1 cup/130 g shelled edamame

¾ cup/115 g finely diced red pepper

¼ cup/10 g basil leaves, roughly chopped and tightly packed

In a small bowl, whisk the shallots, mustard, vinegar and olive oil together. Set aside.

Place the ears of corn in a pot of salted boiling water. Cook for 3 minutes. Drain and cool. Using a chef's knife, strip the kernels from the ears of corn. That should make about 1 cup/130 grams, depending on the size of the ears. Place in a bowl with the farfalle, edamame, red pepper and basil. Toss the ingredients together with ¼ cup/60 milliliters of the reserved vinaigrette.

PER SERVING: Calories 210, protein 7 g, total fat 13 g, carbohydrates 21 g, sodium 65 mg, fiber 3 g

TINA'S TIP: When stripping the corn kernels, don't go too deep or the cob will come off too, and it won't taste very good. Instead, after stripping carefully, turn the knife over and use the dull side to scrape the rest of the corn and the sweet corn juices into the bowl. If you're feeling ambitious, freeze the cobs for the next time you make vegetable stock!

Oui, Oui, MON CHERIE!

NEW POTATOES, OLIVES AND TOMATOES IN A DIJON VINAIGRETTE

While much attention is given to olive oil, I love the zesty flavor and health benefits of olives and I always have assorted varieties in my refrigerator. Mixing them with potatoes may seem to be an unusual combination, but it's a match made in nutrition heaven, and it tastes great! The olives are a very good source of monounsaturated fat, iron, copper and dietary fiber, and the potatoes offer protection against cardiovascular disease and cancer. Serve this Mediterranean-inspired side with grilled or baked chicken, a roast or another hearty entrée. It also travels well and will wow a crowd at a picnic!

YIELD: 8 servings | **TIME:** 35 minutes

2 lb/905 g red-skinned new potatoes, quartered

Salt and freshly ground pepper

2 tbsp/30 ml vegetable oil

¼ cup/65 g prepared olive tapenade or finely chopped Niçoise olives

2 plum tomatoes, seeded and finely chopped

2 tbsp/20 g finely chopped shallot

1 tbsp/11 g Dijon mustard

1 tbsp/15 ml red wine vinegar

¼ cup/60 ml extra-virgin olive oil

2 tbsp/8 g parsley, chopped

Preheat oven to 400°F/200°C or gas mark 6. Place potatoes on a baking sheet. Toss with salt, pepper and vegetable oil and roast for 25 minutes, or until golden and tender when poked with a paring knife.

While the potatoes are roasting, whisk together the olive tapenade, tomatoes, shallot, Dijon, red wine vinegar and extra-virgin olive oil. Reserve.

When potatoes are done, toss with the olive vinaigrette. Adjust seasoning with salt and pepper. Toss with parsley.

PER SERVING: Calories 200, total fat 11 g, protein 3 g, carbohydrates 21 g, sodium 90 mg, fiber 2 g

TINA'S TIP: Try roasting a few different vegetables such as carrots, parsnips or butternut squash along with the potatoes.

The **TAHINI THRILL**

GRILLED EGGPLANT WITH OLIVE OIL, LEMON, TAHINI AND MINT

Tahini paste is a rich, creamy nut butter that's made with ground sesame seeds. It's packed with flavor and nutrition and loaded with phytosterols, a natural compound in the seed, which can help lower cholesterol. Best of all, tahini paste makes everything taste great! While eggplant is a subtle-tasting vegetable, the addition of tahini gives it a rich flavor that's made even more satisfying with a dash of some fresh herbs and spices.

YIELD: 12 servings | **TIME:** 25 minutes

1 large eggplant, cut into 12 slices

2 tbsp/30 ml vegetable oil

¾ tsp salt

2 tbsp/30 g tahini

1 tbsp/15 ml lemon juice

3 tbsp/45 ml hot water

1 tsp/2.5 g ground cumin

½ tsp honey

1 large clove garlic, grated

1 tbsp/4 g parsley, roughly chopped

3 tbsp/18 g mint, thinly sliced

Preheat a grill pan over medium-high heat. Place the eggplant slices on a baking sheet. Using a pastry brush, brush one side of the eggplant with half the oil and sprinkle with ¼ teaspoon of the salt. Turn over and repeat on the second side. Working in batches, place the eggplant on the grill and cook until it begins to soften and grill marks form, about 2 ½ minutes. Turn the eggplant and do the same on the second side. Continue to grill remaining eggplant. As it comes off the grill, stack the eggplant in piles of 4; this will help continue to soften the eggplant and keep it warm.

To make the tahini dressing, combine the tahini, lemon juice, hot water, cumin, honey, garlic and remaining ¼ teaspoon salt. Arrange the eggplant on a platter, drizzle with the dressing and sprinkle with the parsley and mint.

If you have leftovers and want to warm them up, just place the eggplant slices in an oven preheated to 375°F/190°C or gas mark 5 for 5 minutes.

PER SERVING: Calories 45, protein 1 g, total fat 4 g, carbohydrates 3 g, sodium 150 mg, fiber 1 g

TINA'S TIP: This dressing is also incredible on salads. Try grating a little ginger into it for some extra zing!

Not **MEAN GREENS**

GARLIC-SAUTÉED GREENS

If there's one ingredient you always have in your refrigerator, make it lemons. They're incredibly versatile, and the lemon zest adds "brightness" to a dish, while enhancing flavor and aroma. Because the fragrant essential oils of the lemon are in the skin, lemon zest makes vegetables that much more delicious! It does that very thing to kale, and I'm sure it's why my family enjoys kale prepared this way. Topped with crunchy almonds, this recipe explodes with flavor and nutrients to help fight heart disease and cancer.

YIELD: 6 servings | **TIME:** 15 minutes

1 bunch Tuscan kale, tough stems removed and sliced into ½"/1.3 cm strips

2 tbsp/30 ml extra-virgin olive oil

2 cloves garlic, finely chopped

¼ tsp lemon zest

2 tbsp/14 g slivered almonds, toasted

Salt and freshly ground pepper

Bring a large pot of salted water to a boil over high heat. Add the Tuscan kale and simmer until tender, about 5 minutes, depending on how mature the kale is. Drain the kale in a colander and set aside. Place the pot back on the stove over medium heat. Add the olive oil and garlic and, as soon as the garlic starts to sizzle and a couple of pieces start to brown, add the kale and toss it with the garlic and olive oil. Remove from heat, and add the lemon zest and almonds. Toss gently to combine. Taste, and season with salt and pepper.

PER SERVING: Calories 80, protein 2 g, total fat 6 g, carbohydrates 5 g, sodium 15 mg, fiber 1 g

TINA'S TIP: Don't have almonds on hand? Try toasted walnuts, pine nuts or pecans.

Mixed **BAG**

ARUGULA, PEACHES, GORGONZOLA, VIDALIA ONIONS, GREEN BEANS AND WHOLE WHEAT COUSCOUS

The Chinese concept of "yin" and "yang" is used to describe how polar opposites create harmony, and if there were ever a recipe that embodied this philosophy, this is it. The tangy balsamic vinegar balances the sweetness of the peaches. Peppery arugula is tempered by earthly olive oil, and creamy Gorgonzola is perfectly complemented by the crunch of walnuts. It almost tastes too good to be healthy!

YIELD: 4 servings | **TIME:** 35 minutes

2 tsp/10 ml balsamic vinegar

½ tsp Dijon mustard

3 tbsp/45 ml extra-virgin olive oil

1 clove garlic, smashed

½ cup/88 g whole wheat couscous

½ cup/50 g thin green beans

4 cups/268 g baby arugula

½ cup/80 g very thinly sliced Vidalia onion

1 cup/170 g pitted and thinly sliced peach

¼ cup/30 g crumbled Gorgonzola

In a small bowl, combine the balsamic vinegar and Dijon mustard. Slowly whisk in the olive oil and then stir in the garlic. Set aside.

Cook the couscous according to package directions. Allow to cool, about 15 minutes. Bring a small saucepan with salted water to a boil over high heat. Boil the green beans until crisp-tender, about 3 minutes, depending on how thin the beans are. Rinse under cold water until beans are cool to the touch.

To assemble the salad, toss the arugula, Vidalia onion, peach, Gorgonzola, beans and couscous with the vinaigrette. Divide among 4 salad plates.

PER SERVING: Calories 280, protein 8 g, total fat 16 g, carbohydrates 30 g, sodium 220 mg, fiber 5 g

TINA'S TIP: Toasted hazelnuts, walnuts or any other favorite nut would be a nice topping for extra crunch and protein!

Quinoa **TABBOULEH**

QUINOA WITH OLIVE OIL, MINT, PARSLEY AND LEMON

Tabbouleh—a delicious mixture of bulgur and chopped herbs and spices—is the national dish of Lebanon. It is commonly eaten as an appetizer, salad or mezze—one of many small dishes that complement each other. In this recipe, I took some creative liberties and used quinoa instead of bulgur, and the result is a dish that has a satisfying crunch and great taste! Each serving provides 20 percent of a day's worth of vitamin A and 30 percent of your daily vitamin C needs. The fat is of the heart-healthy variety, and the dish is wonderful served warm or chilled.

YIELD: 10 servings | **TIME:** 40 minutes

¾ cup/128 g quinoa

2 cups/470 ml water

1 cup/120 g finely diced cucumber

1 cup/60 g parsley, roughly chopped

½ cup/48 g mint, finely chopped

2 plum tomatoes, chopped

¼ cup/25 g chopped black olives

1 clove garlic, grated

Zest of 1 lemon

3 tbsp/45 ml lemon juice

¼ cup/60 ml extra-virgin olive oil

Salt and freshly ground pepper

In a small saucepan, rinse quinoa until the water runs clear. Place the saucepan on high heat until any remaining water has evaporated and the quinoa begins to pop and crackle, about 3 minutes. Add the water and simmer until the liquid has evaporated and the quinoa is soft, about 20 minutes. Cool completely before adding remaining ingredients to the quinoa. Toss well. Add salt and pepper to taste.

PER SERVING: Calories 120, protein 3 g, total fat 7 g, carbohydrates 12 g, sodium 65 mg, fiber 2 g

TINA'S TIP: Try adding grilled shrimp with or without diced avocado to make this recipe even more delicious!

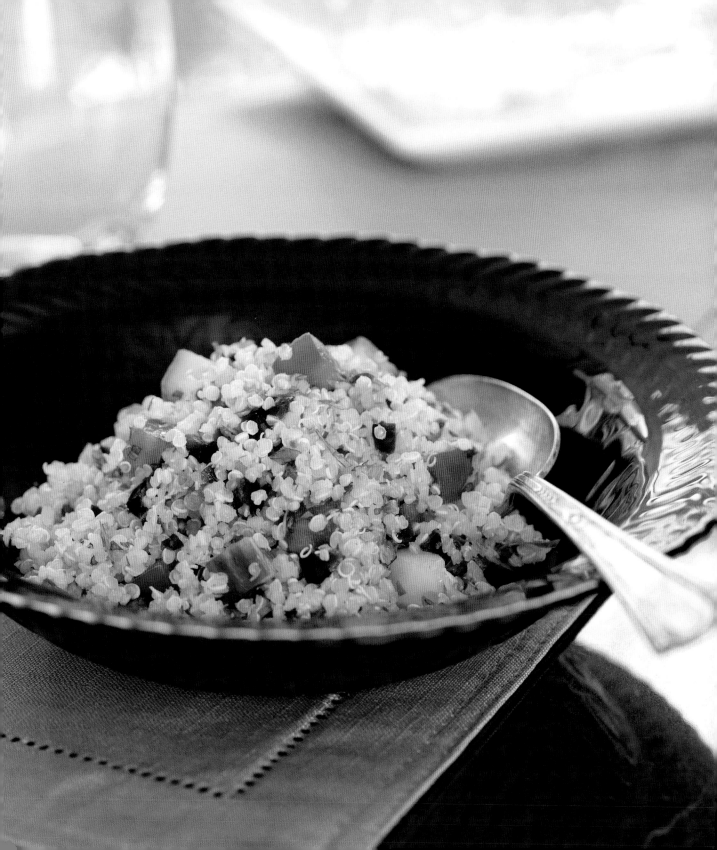

Farmer's HARVEST

MIXED GREENS, SWEET CORN, ZUCCHINI, YELLOW SQUASH, CHERRY TOMATOES AND TOASTED ALMONDS

When summertime deliveries from your community market overwhelm your kitchen or your garden produces more than you know what to do with, it's time to whip out this recipe. Tender summer squash, plump tomatoes and corn from the cob make this a signature summer dish my family looks forward to. For some reason, enjoying it al fresco makes it taste even better! Both the olive oil and the almonds make this salad rich in heart-healthy fat, and the mint leaves provide a beautiful "pop" of color and fresh aroma.

YIELD: 4 servings | **TIME:** 25 minutes

1 tbsp/15 ml balsamic vinegar

½ tsp Dijon mustard

3 tbsp/45 ml extra-virgin olive oil

1 clove garlic, smashed

1 zucchini, cut on the diagonal into 12 slices

1 yellow squash, cut on the diagonal into 12 slices

2 tsp/10 ml vegetable oil

Salt and freshly ground pepper

1 ear corn, husk and silks removed

4 cups/268 g mesclun

½ cup/75 g halved cherry or grape tomatoes

2 tbsp/14 g slivered almonds, toasted

4 mint leaves, finely chopped or chiffonade (see tip)

In a small bowl, combine the balsamic vinegar and Dijon mustard. Slowly whisk in the olive oil and then stir in the garlic. Set aside.

Heat a grill pan over high heat. Spread the zucchini and yellow squash out on a plate or baking tray. Using a pastry brush, lightly brush the zucchini and yellow squash on both sides with vegetable oil. Sprinkle with a small amount of salt and freshly ground pepper. Oil and season the corn as well. When the pan is hot, grill the zucchini and yellow squash for about 1 minute per side, or until nice grill marks appear and they soften slightly. Transfer to the baking tray and reserve. Grill the corn, turning it as grill marks appear, until the whole ear is nicely marked. Allow to cool until it's just warm to the touch. Using a chef's knife, strip the kernels from the ear of corn. The yield should be about ½ cup/75 grams, depending on the size of the ear.

To assemble the salad, place 3 zucchini slices and 3 yellow squash slices on each of 4 plates in a pretty pattern like spokes on a wheel. Toss the mixed greens with the vinaigrette. Place in the middle of each plate so the zucchini and yellow squash peek out. Sprinkle the corn, tomatoes, almonds and mint over the salads.

PER SERVING: Calories 190, protein 6 g, total fat 13 g, carbohydrates 15 g, sodium 30 mg, fiber 3 g

TINA'S TIP: Chiffonade is a method of slicing leaves (mint and basil are good candidates for this), so they end up in fine slices. This looks gorgeous and it also keeps the leaves from oxidizing and turning black. Stack the leaves on top of one another, then very finely slice them.

"Belgian" **SLAW**

BRUSSELS SPROUT SLAW

Brussels sprouts are the unsung heroes of the produce category. The cancer-protective effects we get from this miniature cabbage are related to their very high levels of special phytochemicals. Brussels sprouts also help the body detoxify, and they've been shown to prevent inflammation while offering heart-health benefits. Not a Brussels sprouts fan? This recipe will change your mind, and it just may convert the kids. The addition of grated cheese gives this slaw unbelievable flavor you won't find in any other recipe. Crisp and refreshing, this slaw will surprise you!

YIELD: 4 servings | **TIME:** 40 minutes

3 tbsp/45 ml lemon juice

1 tbsp/15 ml extra-virgin olive oil

¾ tsp salt

8 oz/224 g Brussels sprouts

1 cup/160 g thinly sliced red onion

1 cup/110 g julienned tart apple
(such as Granny Smith)

¼ cup/15 g parsley, chopped

2 tbsp/5 g basil, chopped

½ cup/50 g finely grated
Parmigiano-Reggiano

Freshly ground pepper

Whisk together the lemon juice, olive oil and salt. Set aside.

Remove any brown or yellow leaves from the Brussels sprouts. If the sprouts are very fresh, there won't be discoloration, and you'll have very little waste. Cut the sprouts in half lengthwise. Place the flat side down and slice them as thinly as possible crosswise. Place in a bowl with the onion, apple, parsley, basil and Parmigiano-Reggiano. Toss with vinaigrette. Let sit 15 minutes. Toss again. Taste, adding salt and pepper as desired.

PER SERVING: Calories 140, protein 8 g, total fat 8 g, carbohydrates 12 g, sodium 560 mg, fiber 3 g

TINA'S TIP: Try adding toasted nuts or seeds to the slaw and other herbs like dill and cilantro for a different flavor twist.

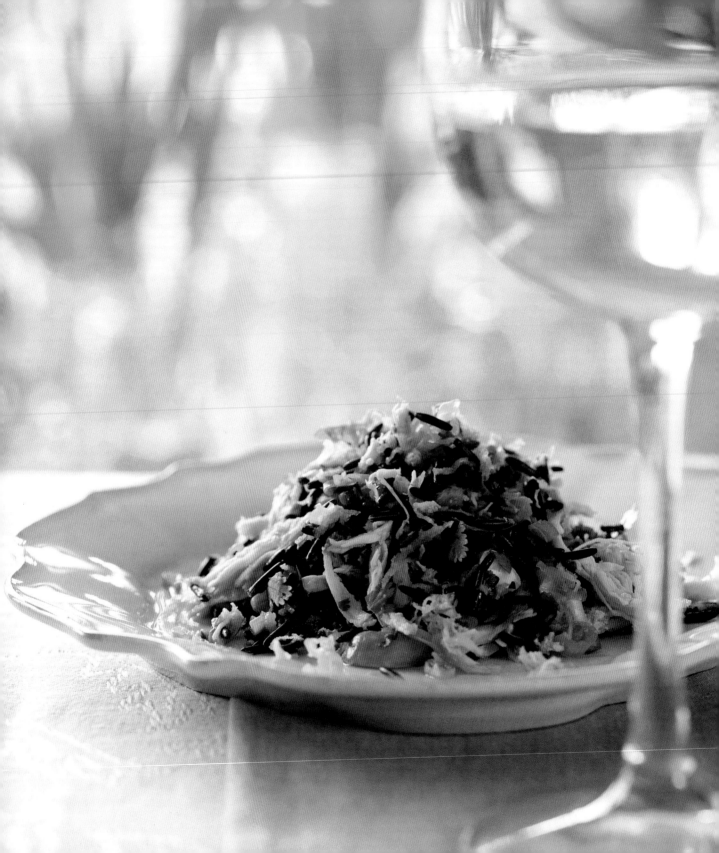

Star-Studded **BLACK RICE**

BLACK RICE SALAD WITH CARROTS, SCALLIONS, CILANTRO, SHREDDED CHICKEN, CASHEWS AND GINGER DRESSING

Black rice is as distinctive as it is delicious. Rich in pigments called anthocyanins, black rice has been linked to decreased risks of cancer and heart disease and improvements in memory and performance. Best of all, it's a versatile ingredient that can be served hot or chilled and used in everything from risotto to pudding. This rice salad is stunningly beautiful, chewy, and satisfying and provides 70 percent of a day's worth of vitamin A along with lots of heart-healthy fats.

YIELD: 4 servings | **TIME**: 45 minutes

⅓ cup/53 g black rice

1 cup/240 ml plus 2 tbsp/30 ml water, divided

⅛ tsp salt

3 tbsp/38 g sugar

3 tbsp/45 ml lime juice

2 tbsp/30 ml Thai fish sauce

1 tsp/5 ml sriracha sauce

1 tsp/3 g grated or finely chopped garlic

1 tbsp/15 ml ginger, grated

½ cup/65 g grated or julienned carrot

2 tbsp/2 g cilantro, roughly chopped

¾ cup/75 g thinly sliced scallion

4 oz/112 g cooked chicken breast, shredded

2 oz/56 g Boston or other leaf lettuce, torn into bite-size pieces

¼ cup/25 g cashews

Place the rice in a small saucepan with 1 cup/235 milliliters of the water and salt. Simmer until the rice is al dente, about 40 minutes. Drain and cool. There should be about 1 cup/165 grams.

While the rice is cooking, make the dressing and prepare the remaining ingredients. Whisk together the sugar, lime juice, fish sauce, remaining 2 tablespoons/30 milliliters water, sriracha sauce, garlic and ginger. Reserve.

To assemble the salad, place the carrots, cilantro, scallions, chicken, lettuce and rice in a bowl. Toss with 5 tablespoons/75 milliliters of the dressing. Divide among 4 salad plates and sprinkle with the cashews.

PER SERVING: Calories 250, protein 9 g, total fat 10 g, carbohydrates 35 g, sodium 850 mg, fiber 3 g

TINA'S TIP: If you can't find black rice, try brown basmati rice instead.

Veggie NICE SALAD

MIXED GREENS WITH GRAPEFRUIT, BEETS, RICOTTA SALATA, RED ONION AND BASIL

Contrary to popular belief, fat doesn't make you fat and is not the sole reason for heart disease or the obesity crisis. Honestly, fat is my secret to staying slim! Eaten wisely, fat is delicious and nutritious; it's essential to absorbing fat-soluble vitamins and keeps you full and content. In this recipe, the addition of olive oil and cheese to sweet grapefruit segments makes the salad hearty and refreshing at the same time. It also delivers 60 percent of a day's worth of vitamin C, 25 percent of your daily vitamin A needs, 15 percent of your calcium requirements, and yes, a good dose of heart-healthy fat.

YIELD: 4 servings | **TIME:** 40 minutes

4 oz/113 g beets

1 tbsp/15 ml balsamic vinegar

½ tsp Dijon mustard

3 tbsp/45 ml extra-virgin olive oil

1 clove garlic, smashed

4 cups/220 g mesclun

¼ cup/10 g basil leaves, shredded

2 oz/56 g very thinly sliced red onion

12 oz/340 g pink grapefruit segments

3 oz/84 g ricotta salata, crumbled

Place the beets in a saucepan of salted water. Boil until a knife can easily be inserted into the beets, about 30 minutes depending on size of beets. Allow to cool in cold water. Peel the beets and cut into bite-size segments.

In a small bowl, combine the balsamic vinegar and Dijon mustard. Slowly whisk in the olive oil and then stir in the garlic. Set aside.

To assemble the salad, toss the mesclun, basil and red onion with 3 tablespoons/ 45 milliliters of the vinaigrette. Divide among 4 salad plates. Divide the grapefruit segments and ricotta salata among the plates.

PER SERVING: Calories 200, protein 6 g, total fat 14 g, carbohydrates 13 g, sodium 340 mg, fiber 3 g

TINA'S TIP: If ricotta salata isn't available, try using low-fat feta cheese or queso for a nice tangy alternative.

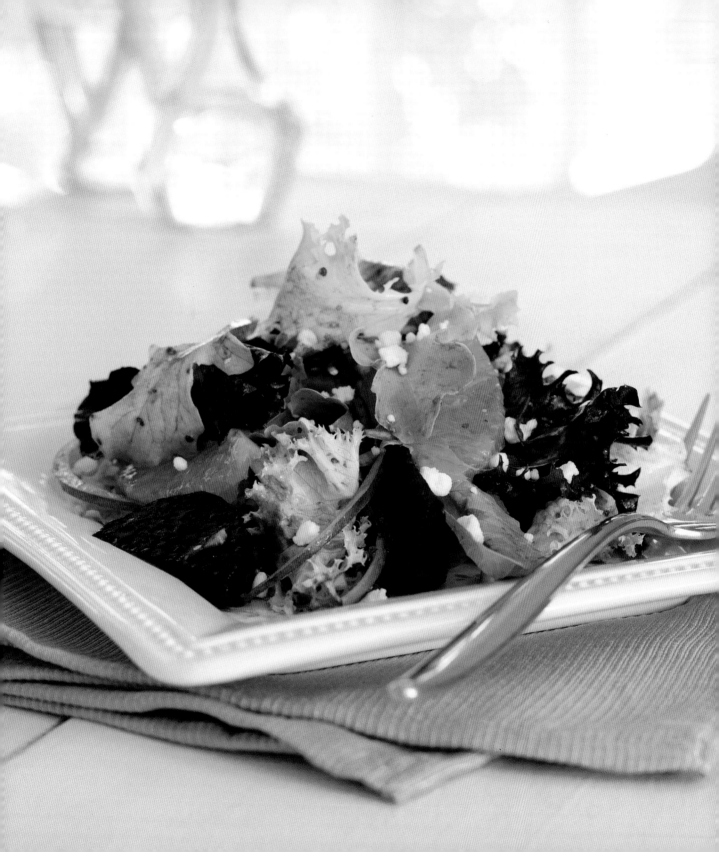

Tina's **FAMOUS FARRO**

FARRO WITH ROASTED BUTTERNUT SQUASH, SWISS CHARD, WALNUTS AND DRIED CRANBERRIES

Emmer, or farro as it's called in Italy, is an ancient ancestor of wheat. If you've never eaten farro, you'll soon make it a pantry staple; it's satisfying, nutritious, inexpensive and versatile. I use it in soup, salads, stuffing and pilafs. You can even bake with it. New science shows that farro is a rich source of disease-fighting antioxidants. In this recipe, each serving provides 120 percent of a day's worth of vitamin A and more than one-third of your daily requirement for vitamin C.

YIELD: 8 servings | **TIME:** 30 minutes

½ **small butternut squash, washed, peeled and cut into ½"/1.3 cm cubes (about 1 ¼ cups/195 g)**

Salt and freshly ground pepper

1 tbsp/15 ml vegetable oil

1 cup/200 g pearled farro

1 tbsp/15 ml extra-virgin olive oil, plus extra for drizzling (optional)

2 tbsp/30 ml red wine vinegar

1 clove garlic, finely chopped or grated

8 oz/230 g Swiss chard, sliced into ¼"/6 mm ribbons

½ **cup/55 g chopped walnuts**

½ **cup/60 g dried cranberries, unsweetened**

½ **cup/30 g parsley, roughly chopped**

Preheat oven to 400°F/200°F or gas mark 6. Place the butternut squash on a baking sheet and toss with salt, pepper and vegetable oil. Roast, turning the chunks over once or twice, until soft and golden, about 20 minutes.

Place the farro in a pot of salted water and bring to a boil over high heat; cook until al dente, about 15 minutes. Drain.

While the farro is cooking, whisk together the olive oil, red wine vinegar and garlic. Stir half into the farro while it is warm. Reserve the rest. Allow the farro to cool to room temperature.

Place the Swiss chard in a saucepan. If it is still wet from washing, cover the pot and heat to wilt the leaves and cook the stems, about 5 minutes. If the leaves are dry, add a couple of tablespoons of water to the pan before proceeding. Drain any excess liquid from the pan.

Add the butternut squash, Swiss chard, walnuts, cranberries, parsley, and remaining oil and vinegar to the farro. Stir to combine. Taste and adjust seasoning with salt and pepper. Drizzle with additional olive oil, if desired.

PER SERVING: Calories 210, protein 5 g, total fat 9 g, carbohydrates 32 g, sodium 65 mg, fiber 6 g

TINA'S TIP: Don't be intimidated by that squash! The secret to cutting squash effectively is to always keep the tip of the blade on the cutting board and secure the blade of your knife into the flesh of the squash. Press down carefully, never letting the knife come off the cutting board. The leverage makes it simple to cut the squash into chunks.

SIESTA Special

CHILLED RICE SALAD WITH AVOCADO, TOMATOES AND BLACK BEANS

Who says white rice isn't healthy? Just look at the nutrient profile of this dish, and you'll surely change your mind. This chilled rice salad is chockfull of veggies, loaded with flavor, and a nice source of fiber and contributes valuable heart-healthy fats to the diet. Plus, it looks beautiful on the table! In particular, this dish is a favorite among the teenage girls in my household because, I am told, "It makes us feel healthy!" Who can argue with that? When you purchase the sun-dried tomatoes, choose those packed in olive oil, because you'll use the oil in the recipe. The rice salad will last 3 days in the refrigerator and makes a delicious lunch or summery dinner.

YIELD: 5 servings | **TIME:** 40 minutes

1 cup/195 g raw white rice

2 cups/470 ml water

1 (15 ½ oz/434 g) can black beans, rinsed and drained

¼ cup/28 g chopped sun-dried tomatoes in olive oil (oil reserved for later use)

½ cup/75 g diced red pepper

1 cup/145 g diced avocado (about 1 avocado)

½ cup/8 g cilantro leaves, washed, dried and coarsely chopped

¼ tsp kosher salt

2 tsp/5 g chia seeds

2 tbsp/30 ml lemon juice

2 tbsp/30 ml reserved sun-dried tomato oil (or extra-virgin olive oil)

In a medium pot, place rice and water, warming over high heat until water boils. Cover, reduce heat to low, and cook rice for 20 minutes. Remove from heat, and let rice sit 10 minutes.

Meanwhile, in a large bowl, add black beans, sun-dried tomatoes, red pepper, avocado and cilantro. When ready, add rice to a colander and rinse with cold water to remove starchiness from rice. Add rinsed rice to the bowl, and mix with ingredients.

In a small bowl, combine salt, chia seeds, lemon juice and sun-dried tomato oil. Pour dressing over salad, stirring to combine. Taste, and season with more lemon juice or sun-dried tomato oil, if needed.

PER SERVING: Calories 180, protein 7 g, total fat 6 g, carbohydrates 27 g, sodium 160 mg, fiber 8 g

TINA'S TIP: If you wish, brown rice can be used in place of the white rice. Any leftover vegetables you have in the refrigerator can also be used in this salad. Try scallions, carrots and cucumbers.

Heart **THROB**

KALE SALAD WITH DRIED CHERRIES, WALNUTS AND WARM ANCHOVY DRESSING

Most likely, if you open a can of anchovies, you're going to hear squeals and jeers from those around you—adults included. However, those same people will gladly use Worcestershire sauce and green goddess dressing and eat Caesar salad, each of which incorporates anchovies. Perhaps the visual of the little filets in the can aren't appealing, but what's so different about anchovies from the fish you buy at the market? One's packed in oil and the other in ice. My response to the fuss? Get over it! Anchovies are delicious, and one of my secret ingredients to making meals taste incredible, this kale salad included. After one bite, you will be addicted. The warm anchovy dressing wilts the kale, so it's tender yet still crisp; the nuts give the salad a nice crunch; and the cherries offer a bit of sweetness. Best of all, this salad is extraordinarily good for heart health. More than 60 percent of the fat is mono- and polyunsaturated. Plus, you get 120 percent of a day's worth of vitamin A and 80 percent of your vitamin C needs in just one serving.

YIELD: 6 servings | **TIME:** 30 minutes

1 bunch kale

⅓ cup/35 g chopped walnuts

¼ cup/30 g dried cherries

¼ cup/60 ml extra-virgin olive oil

½ tsp crushed red pepper flakes

½ (2 oz/56 g) tin flat anchovy filets

1½ tbsp/22.5 ml lemon juice

To prepare kale, remove the kale leaves from the stem, discarding stems. Layer a few kale leaves on top of each other, roll into a circular shape and thinly slice to julienne. Place chopped kale into a large bowl. Top with walnuts and dried cherries.

In a heavy-duty small pot over medium-high heat, add olive oil, red pepper flakes and anchovies. Very carefully, whisk until anchovies are dissolved, just 30 seconds to 1 minute. Remove from heat, and quickly add lemon juice. (Be careful. It will sizzle, so step back!) Pour dressing in increments over kale salad, tossing to incorporate. Serve.

PER SERVING: Calories 180, protein 5 g, total fat 15 g, carbohydrates 9 g, sodium 360 mg, fiber 1 g

TINA'S TIP: The most time-consuming part of this recipe is cleaning and chopping the kale, which can be done in advance of dinner. Be sure to use a salad spinner to dry the kale the best you can. The drier the kale, the better the dressing can cling to it. Also, dried cranberries can be used in place of the cherries.

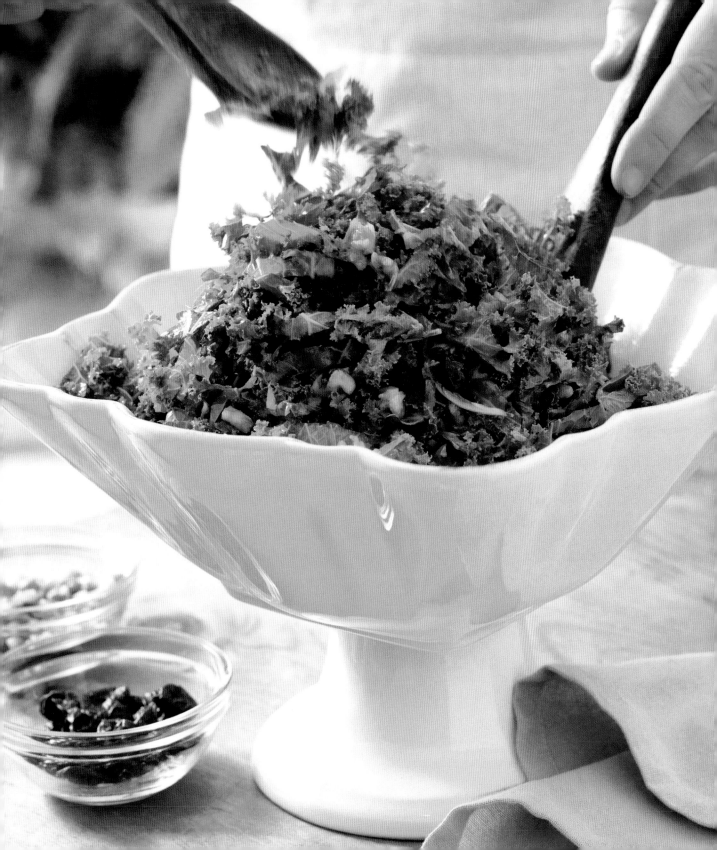

YAM, YAM Good!

HONEYED MASHED YAMS WITH PUMPKIN SEEDS

Most people think yams and sweet potatoes are related, but they're not. Yams are grown in Africa, Asia and Latin America and are sweeter than sweet potatoes. While yams are not as popular as sweet potatoes, they're slowly becoming more available Stateside. Even though it might be a bit more challenging to seek out yams, it's worth it; they are a wonderfully rich source of vitamins A, C and B complex, and they are loaded with potassium, calcium and iron, minerals essential to good health at all stages of life. This mashed potato recipe is beloved by toddlers and teens alike. Younger children won't care for the scallions, so use them as a garnish on the adults' portions.

YIELD: 6 servings | **TIME:** 25 minutes

2 lb/905 g yams, peeled and diced

1 tbsp/15 ml reduced-sodium soy sauce

1½ tbsp/22.5 ml honey

1½ tbsp/21 g unsalted butter

½ cup/120 ml whole milk

2 tbsp/12 g chopped scallion

¼ cup/34 g salted, roasted pepita seeds

In a large, heavy-duty pot, add chopped yams, and cover with water. Bring to a boil over high heat, and cook until a fork or knife inserted into yams doesn't meet any resistance, about 10 minutes. Drain water from yams in a colander. Transfer cooked yams to a food processor. Add soy sauce, honey and butter. Purée yams, pouring the milk through the feeder tube of food processor as it processes, and combine until yams form a smooth texture. (Note that you may need to use a spatula to scrape down mixture in the food processor bowl.) Transfer yam purée to a large bowl, and stir in scallions and pepita seeds. Serve.

PER SERVING: Calories 200, protein 4 g, total fat 5 g, carbohydrates 36 g, sodium 70 mg, fiber 5 g

TINA'S TIP: In this recipe, sweet potatoes can't be substituted for yams. Look for true yams in international or Latin markets.

OODLES OF NOODLES Salad

CHILLED NOODLE SALAD WITH PEANUT DRESSING

Making a commitment to healthy eating is easy. Following through on any given day is what's tough! Lack of time, ideas or ingredients will challenge you, but this recipe is one you can whip up in minutes, because it relies on pantry staples, condiments and veggies you have on hand. If you don't have soba noodles, use thin, whole wheat spaghetti; if you don't have sriracha sauce, use another type of hot sauce—or don't use it at all if your family prefers milder flavors. Broccoli, green peppers, mushrooms, bok choy and frozen, thawed snow peas can work, too. Your options are endless! Best of all, this creamy, peanut-y flavored, chilled salad is an effective way to coax kids to eat their vegetables. This salad is delicious for lunch or dinner on a warm summer evening, and it's rich in heart-healthy mono- and polyunsaturated fats.

YIELD: 6 servings | **TIME:** 30 minutes

¼ cup/65 g chunky natural peanut butter

¼ cup/60 g tahini

1 tbsp/15 ml reduced-sodium soy sauce

1 tbsp/15 ml sesame oil

1 tbsp/15 ml sriracha

1 tbsp/15 ml rice vinegar

2 tsp/10 ml honey

2 tsp/5 g grated ginger

¼ cup/60 ml water

½ cup/40 g julienned snow peas

6 oz/170 g soba noodles

1 cup/100 g thinly sliced scallion

1 cup/120 g diced cucumber

½ cup/55 g grated carrot

1 cup/150 g julienned red pepper

2 tsp/5 g black and white sesame seeds, toasted (optional)

Combine the peanut butter, tahini, soy sauce, sesame oil, sriracha, rice vinegar, honey, ginger and water in a small saucepan. Heat over low heat and stir just to combine. Turn off heat and reserve.

Bring a large pot of salted water to a boil over high heat. Cook the snow peas until bright green and crisp, about 30 seconds. Remove snow peas (do not drain) and run under cold water to stop the cooking. Use the same water to cook the noodles to al dente according to package directions. Drain and run under cold water to stop the cooking. Toss the noodles with the snow peas, scallion, cucumber, carrot, pepper and reserved sauce. Sprinkle with the sesame seeds, if using.

PER SERVING: Calories 270, protein 9 g, total fat 14 g, carbohydrates 30 g, sodium 170 mg, fiber 4 g

TINA'S TIP: Tahini and nut butters last for months in the refrigerator, even after being opened. Stock up to have them on hand for everything from hummus to salad dressing.

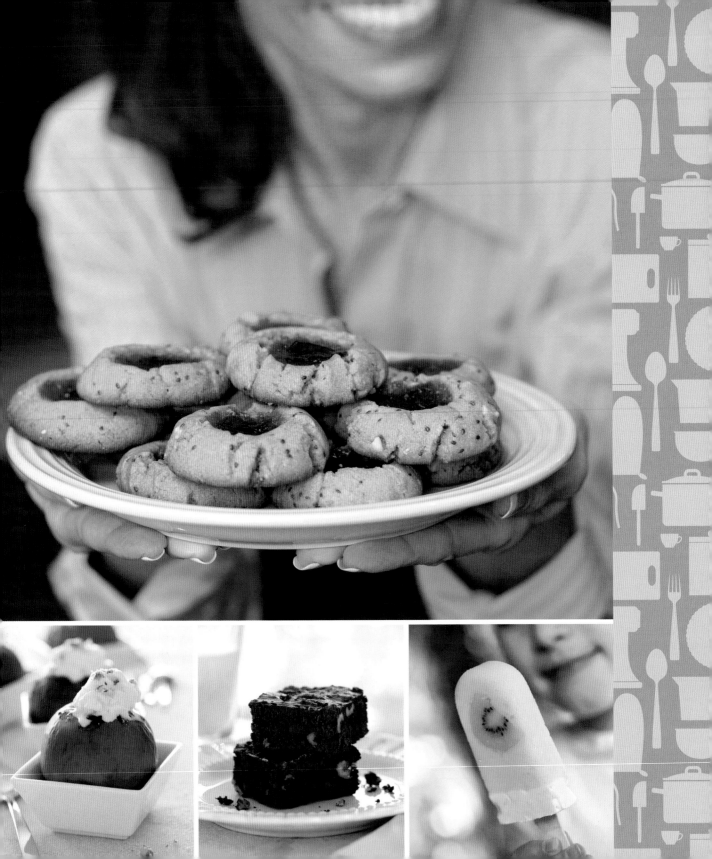

Sweet Surprises

Save room for dessert! Guilt-free treats make happy endings!

I come from a long line of bakers who made Italian delicacies, including torrone, zeppole and sfogliatini. If you're not familiar with these pastries, all you need to know is that consumption of these babies will have the scale tipping in the wrong direction in no time.

When I began to bake on my own, experimenting with different ingredients and techniques, I realized that dessert doesn't need to be ultra-caloric to be satisfying and memorable. All you need is flavor—not necessarily fat—to make unforgettable, seemingly indulgent desserts.

On the next few pages, you'll find recipes for sweet endings that will satisfy your craving for something yummy without sabotaging your weight, because the flavors in my recipes come from fruit, herbs and spices. Not only are these desserts sweet and skinny, but they also contribute nutrients to your diet. Not one recipe has empty calories, so each treat can be part of your family's healthy lifestyle.

Every delicious dessert can be made quickly, and there's something for everyone! Hosting a party? My Skinny Cheesecake Minis fit the bill. Need to wow the in-laws with something special? Whip up my Angel's Slice. Want an everyday treat that's also perfect for a snack? Double Dippin' Delights are the answer. No one will ever know these desserts are light, and best of all, you'll enjoy making, serving and eating these guilt-free goodies.

Remember, always save room for dessert!

Skinny
CHEESECAKE MINIS

NO-BAKE INDIVIDUAL CHEESECAKES WITH RASPBERRY DRIZZLE

I love decadent desserts and gravitate to anything that's creamy, chocolaty or gooey. To have my cake and eat it too, I made the classic cheesecake recipe slimmer and trimmer but just as satisfying. Considering a slice of regular cheesecake can have between 400 and 1,150 calories, my skinny, crowd-pleasing cheesecake is guilt-free! Best of all, new research shows that cheese contains a unique form of fat that may be absorbed differently than fat from other foods, suggesting a favorable effect on heart health. Dairy food has also shown the ability to lower blood pressure and decrease overall weight. The kids will love having their own personal dessert. My lighter version doesn't require baking, can be done in a pinch, and looks beautiful drizzled with a bit of raspberry coulis.

YIELD: 4 servings | **TIME:** 30 minutes plus chilling time

Special equipment: 4 (4 oz/120 ml) ramekins or custard cups

8 oz/240 g low fat cream cheese, at room temperature

½ cup/112 g low fat sour cream, at room temperature

⅔ cup/80 g confectioner's sugar, sifted

¼ tsp lemon zest

1 tbsp/15 ml lemon juice

2 tsp/10 ml vanilla extract

1 recipe Raspberry Coulis (recipe follows)

4 tsp/8 g graham cracker crumbs

2 tsp/10 g unsalted butter, melted

Dark chocolate, for garnish (optional)

Mint leaves, for garnish (optional)

In the bowl of an electric mixer with the paddle attachment, beat the cream cheese, sour cream, sugar, lemon zest, lemon juice and vanilla until smooth. Tear 2 paper towels in half, lengthwise. You will have 4 pieces of paper towel. Wet each piece, and then squeeze out any excess water. Line the ramekins so the excess paper towel hangs over the edge. Divide the cream cheese mixture among the ramekins. Knock them on the counter to get rid of any air pockets. Fold the paper towels over the cream cheese mixture so they are pressed onto the surface. Refrigerate for 2 to 24 hours. While the cheesecakes are setting, make the berry coulis.

After chilling, pull the paper towels from the surface of the cheesecakes. Combine the graham cracker crumbs and melted butter. Divide the mixture among the ramekins, and spread the mixture to form a "crust." Press it gently into the cheesecakes. Unmold onto plates, graham cracker side down, and serve with 2 tablespoons/30 milliliters of berry coulis on each cake. Garnish with shavings of dark chocolate and a mint leaf, if desired.

PER SERVING: Calories 250, protein 6 g, total fat 11 g, carbohydrates 31 g, sodium 300 mg, fiber 0 g

TINA'S TIP: If you forget to bring the cream cheese and sour cream to room temperature, microwave them on low power, stirring occasionally to keep any hot spots from forming.

Raspberry COULIS

Raspberries tend to go bad very quickly, so try to use them within a day or so. Swish them gently in cold water, just before you use them, as opposed to after you buy them and before putting them in the refrigerator. This will help preserve their longevity; moisture on their delicate skin hastens spoilage.

YIELD: 1 ½ cups/350 ml | **TIME:** 10 minutes

1 (12 oz/336 g) bag frozen berries (NOT in sauce), defrosted

2 tbsp/25 g sugar

2 tsp/10 ml lemon juice, or more to taste

3 to 4 tbsp/45 to 60 ml water

Place the thawed berries in a blender with the sugar and lemon juice. Purée until smooth, adding water to achieve the desired consistency, and the sugar is dissolved. Can be kept refrigerated for 5 days or frozen for at least 2 months.

PER 1-TABLESPOON/15-MILLILITER SERVING: Calories 5, protein 0 g, total fat 0 g, carbohydrates 1 g, sodium 0 mg, fiber 0 g

TINA'S TIP: This sauce can be made with frozen blackberries, as well. Freeze leftover coulis in ice cube trays. Once frozen, put the cubes into a zip-top bag. Frozen pieces can easily be thawed in the microwave, or toss them into the blender when making smoothies for added nutrition and flavor.

Cozy Comfort
BREAD PUDDING

PEACH, RASPBERRY AND ALMOND BREAD PUDDING

Bread pudding is a classic dessert from years gone by, but its timelessness endures. It has all the elements of decadence; it's buttery, creamy and custardy, and a good bourbon sauce makes it complete. While my father and I would love to eat it every day for dessert, it probably wouldn't be a good idea! So, I created this slimmer version, which will satisfy your craving for the comfort food favorite without packing on the pounds. Raspberries contribute disease-fighting ellagic acid, almonds offer cholesterol-lowering powers, and a generous sprinkling of cinnamon adds brain-boosting powers and a smack of flavor.

YIELD: 8 (4 oz/113 g) ramekins | **TIME:** 45 minutes

3 eggs

1 cup/235 ml skim milk

3 tbsp/36 g sugar

Pinch salt

1 tsp/5 ml vanilla extract

¼ tsp almond extract

6 oz/170 g brioche or challah or white bread, ideally stale or dried out in the oven, cut into 1"/2.5 cm cubes

1 cup/125 g raspberries

1 cup/170 g roughly chopped peaches

¼ cup/28 g. slivered, toasted almonds

Preheat oven to 350°F/180°C or gas mark 4. In a medium bowl, whisk together the eggs, milk, sugar, salt, vanilla and almond extracts. Gently toss in the bread, raspberries and peaches. Divide mixture between 8 (4 oz/113 g) ramekins. Press down slightly. Sprinkle with almonds. Bake for 30 minutes. Allow to cool slightly before serving.

PER SERVING: Calories 150, protein 6 g, total fat 5 g, carbohydrates 22 g, sodium 150 mg, fiber 1 g

TINA'S TIP: Bread pudding is a great way to use all different types of bread, so be creative! You can try different fruit, as well. To dress up this dessert for entertaining, add a splash of raspberry liqueur or peach schnapps to the adults' portions.

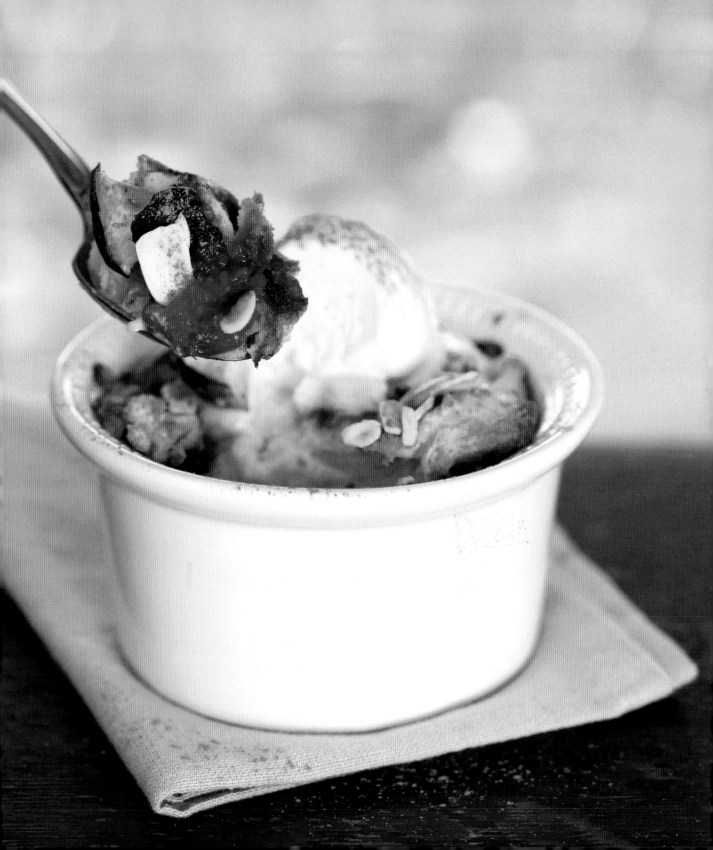

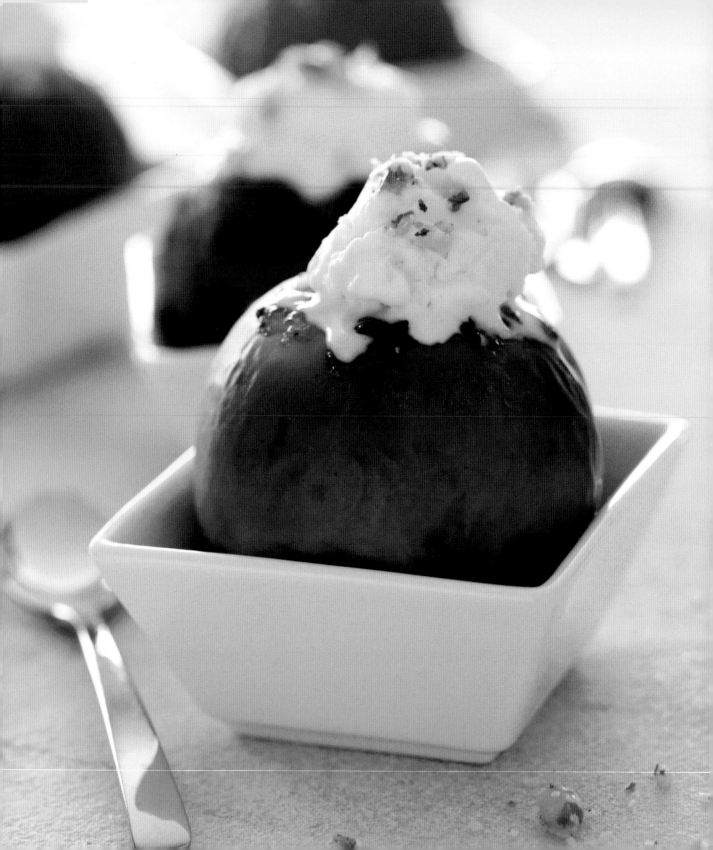

The **APPLE OF MY EYE**

BAKED APPLES WITH CARAMEL, HAZELNUTS AND FROZEN YOGURT

This all-American fruit is a sweet and juicy source of nutrition. Apples are loaded with vitamin C and cancer-fighting polyphenols that work together to keep us healthy. Most people don't realize that they're also a source of amino acids that bolster muscle growth in young and old alike. Baked and filled with sweet preserves, these apples will please the pickiest eaters, especially if they get to fill the apples themselves! And don't limit the fillings to strawberry. Experiment with everything from apricot to quince!

YIELD: 4 servings | **TIME:** 50 minutes

4 Granny Smith or Cortland apples (or other baking variety)

½ cup/160 g strawberry preserves

1 cup/245 g low-fat vanilla frozen yogurt

2 tbsp/14 g roughly chopped toasted hazelnuts

Preheat oven to 350°F/180°C or gas mark 4. Using a paring knife or an apple corer, remove the core of the apples. Use a melon baller or teaspoon to scoop out additional seeds and fibrous core. Place apples on a baking tray. Stuff each apple with 2 tablespoons/30 g preserves. Bake for 40 minutes, or until softened. For each serving, place in a bowl and top with a scoop of frozen yogurt and ½ tablespoon/7 grams hazelnuts.

PER SERVING: Calories 250, protein 5 g, total fat 5 g, carbohydrates 50 g, sodium 45 mg, fiber 2 g

TINA'S TIP: Apples will cook for different lengths of time, depending upon their variety, size and ripeness. So, you'll need to check your baked apples frequently while they cook. The final product should be soft but not mushy.

Whey to Go
YOGURT BRÛLÉE

FRUITED YOGURT BRÛLÉE

This is the easiest dessert I've ever made, and it's hard to believe it's healthy. The brûlée's sweet taste and creamy texture are powerful enough to win over non-yogurt lovers, and the dish is pretty enough to serve for brunch. It provides 80 percent of your daily vitamin C requirement and 11 grams of protein, mostly from whey. Whey is a by-product of making yogurt. It's that watery liquid on top of your yogurt and what you stir into the solid portion, before you eat it. Whey also contributes vitamins and minerals to our diet. Nutrition aside, this dessert is a no-fat taste of heaven!

YIELD: 4 servings | **TIME:** 15 minutes

Special equipment: 4 (6 oz/175 ml) ramekins or custard cups

2 cups/460 g plain nonfat Greek yogurt

3 tbsp/36 g plus 2 tsp/8 g sugar, divided

1 tsp/5 ml vanilla extract, divided

2 cups/250 g raspberries, strawberries, blueberries or other fruit, chopped into bite-size pieces

Dark chocolate, for serving (optional)

4 mint leaves, for garnish (optional)

Place the yogurt in a bowl and stir in 4 teaspoons/16 grams of the sugar and ½ teaspoon/2.5 milliliters of the vanilla. Refrigerate while chopping the fruit. Place the fruit in a bowl with 1 tablespoon/12 grams sugar (perhaps less depending on how sweet the fruit is) and the remaining ½ teaspoon/2.5 milliliters vanilla. Stir without breaking the fruit.

To assemble, place ½ cup/65 grams fruit in the bottom of 4 (6-ounce/175-milliliter) custard cups or ramekins. Spread ½ cup/65 grams of yogurt over the fruit. Brûlées can be refrigerated at this stage for several hours. When ready to serve, sprinkle 1 teaspoon/4 grams of the remaining sugar over each custard cup and place under the broiler for 30 seconds to 1 minute. Watch carefully and remove when sugar has caramelized. Or use a mini blowtorch to achieve the same effect.

Garnish with grated dark chocolate and a fresh mint leaf, if desired.

PER SERVING: Calories 130, protein 11 g, fat 0 g, carbohydrates 23 g, sodium 45 mg, fiber 2 g

TINA'S TIP: Any of your favorite fruits can work with this recipe. Vanilla-flavored yogurt works, too. Or play with adding spices. A dash of coriander is wonderful over fruit!

Over THE RAINBOW

PINEAPPLE, KIWI AND ORANGE ZEST ICE POPS

During the summer when I was a kid, my family would go to the beach and we'd stay all day, swimming, building sandcastles, looking for sea glass, taking long walks, picnicking, digging in the sand and sometimes fishing. By the end of the day, I was spent, and it was with great enthusiasm that I welcomed the ice cream truck, when it pulled into the beach parking lot at four o'clock. I needed energy, I wanted to cool off, and those orange creamsicles were calling my name. Certainly, times have changed, but my memories of those ice-cold and colorful treats remain vivid, and they're the inspiration for this refreshing ice pop recipe. They're easy and fun to make, contain 60 percent of a day's worth of vitamin C, and they'll make kids of all ages very, very happy.

YIELD: 6 ice pops | **TIME:** 10 minutes plus freezing time

2 cups/310 g diced pineapple

2 tbsp/24 g sugar, divided

1 kiwi

6 tbsp/90 g low-fat Greek yogurt

1 tsp/2 g orange zest

Place the pineapple and 1 tablespoon/12 grams of the sugar in a blender and purée until smooth (be sure to completely break down the pineapple or it will have a stringy texture).

Peel the kiwi and slice in half lengthwise, then each half into 6 half-moons.

Place the yogurt, orange zest and remaining 1 tablespoon/12 grams sugar in a bowl and whisk until the sugar has dissolved.

Divide the pineapple mixture among 6 ice pop molds, making sure there's enough room for 1 tablespoon/15 grams of the yogurt mixture. Place 2 pieces of kiwi in each mold, one on each side, and press them against the sides so when it's unmolded the kiwi will show through. Top with 1 tablespoon/15 grams of the yogurt mixture in each mold. Freeze until solid.

PER ICE POP: Calories 60, protein 2 g, total fat 0 g, carbohydrates 13 g, sodium 10 mg, fiber 1 g

TINA'S TIP: Try this trick for peeling a kiwi: Cut both ends off the kiwi. Guide a spoon under the kiwi skin and twist the kiwi and let the spoon peel the kiwi. The skin will slip right off.

Double
DIPPIN' DELIGHTS

DARK CHOCOLATE—DIPPED DRIED APRICOTS WITH HEMP SEED

The use of hemp seeds is slowly but steadily gaining popularity in modern meals, but if you haven't tried them yet, you're in for a treat! Hemp seeds are a complete protein, which contains all ten amino acids. They're also rich in vitamin E and omega-3 fatty acids and have a wonderful nutty taste. Combined with dark chocolate and sweet, dried apricots, they make an incredibly satisfying and healthy dessert that everyone will enjoy. This is also a fun recipe for the kids to help make; dipping the chocolate-covered fruit into the seeds is a great way to get them excited about cooking!

YIELD: 30 pieces | **TIME:** 25 minutes

⅔ cup/64 g hemp seeds

6 oz/170 g dark chocolate, chopped into small pieces

30 dried apricots

Place the hemp seeds into a shallow dish. Prepare a baking sheet by lining it with parchment paper.

Next, create a hot water bath to temper the chocolate by filling a medium pot with a few inches/centimeters of water. Bring to a boil over high heat. Add half of the chopped chocolate into a heatproof bowl. Fit bowl on top of pot. Using a heatproof spatula, stir the chocolate until it completely melts, about 2 to 3 minutes. Carefully remove bowl from water bath. Add remaining chocolate pieces in 2 batches, stirring to combine and melt. Dip each dried apricot into the tempered chocolate to coat three-fourths of the apricot and then dip into the hemp seeds. Place on prepared baking sheet. Repeat, until all dried apricots are coated. Place in the fridge until hardened, up to an hour. Remove from fridge, and store in a sealed container until served.

PER APRICOT: Calories 60, protein 2 g, total fat 3 g carbohydrates 8 g, sodium 0 mg, fiber 1 g

TINA'S TIP: The apricots can also be rolled into chopped nuts or a combination of ground nuts and hemp seeds.

ANGEL'S Slice

CHOCOLATE CHIP ANGEL FOOD CAKE WITH GANACHE

One bite of my guilt-free cake, and you'll understand where its name came from!
This dessert is an all-natural slice of heaven made even more delicious with the addition
of dark chocolate. Just 1 ounce/28 grams of dark chocolate daily can make a significant
contribution to the antioxidant content of your diet. That's not to say that you should binge
on this cake, but a slice now and again won't break your calorie bank and will keep you in
your skinny jeans. The family won't even know it's "healthy." It fires on all cylinders:
it looks decadent, tastes great and will make any occasion festive.

YIELD: 12 servings | **TIME:** 50 minutes

14 tbsp/105 g cake flour

¼ cup/30 g unsweetened cocoa powder

¼ tsp salt

12 large egg whites

1 ¼ cups/250 g sugar

2 tsp/10 ml vanilla extract

10 oz/280 g dark chocolate (70 percent cacao), finely chopped, divided

6 tbsp/90 ml low-fat buttermilk

Preheat oven to 350°F/180°C or gas mark 4.

Whisk together the cake flour, cocoa and salt.

In the bowl of an electric mixer, whip the egg whites on high speed until medium peaks form, about 1 minute. Add the sugar in a steady stream and continue to whip until stiff peaks form, 2 minutes more. Stir in the vanilla. Carefully fold in the dry ingredients and half the chocolate. Pour into a tube pan. Bake for 35 minutes, or until a toothpick inserted near the center comes out clean. Allow to cool.

While the cake is cooking make the ganache. Place the remaining half of the chocolate and buttermilk in a small saucepan. Heat over low heat, stirring until smooth. Add a little water if needed to thin out the sauce to a pourable consistency.

For each serving, drizzle approximately 2 tablespoons/30 milliliters ganache over a slice of cake.

PER SLICE: Calories 250, protein 7 g, total fat 7 g, carbohydrates 44 g, sodium 120 mg, fiber 1 g

TINA'S TIP: When separating eggs, make sure that no yolk gets into the whites or the eggs will not whip. The safest way to do this is to use 2 small bowls. Separate one egg. When the egg white is separated cleanly, move it into the large electric mixer bowl, thereby avoiding the possibility of contaminating the whole batch.

Mighty
MELON-BERRY FLOAT

WATERMELON, STRAWBERRY AND MINT FLOAT

A healthy diet provides essential nutrients at every meal, and dessert is no exception. That's why I try to incorporate fruit, yogurt, dark chocolate or cheese into my sweet endings. As opposed to a milkshake, which contains milk, ice cream and flavorings, a float is made by adding soda or seltzer to ice cream. I've slimmed down this float by using frozen yogurt, and by blending two vitamin C–rich fruits, giving just one serving of this fizzy pink beverage nearly half a day's worth of the immune-boosting vitamin. Kids can even enjoy it for an afternoon treat, and to make a fun, adult beverage, substitute the seltzer with Prosecco!

YIELD: 2 floats | **TIME:** 10 minutes

2 cups/300 g seeded and roughly chopped watermelon, preferably chilled

½ cup/85 g sliced strawberries, preferably chilled

¾ cup/180 ml cold seltzer

6 oz/168 g vanilla frozen yogurt

4 mint leaves, sliced

Place the watermelon and strawberries in a blender or food processor and process until smooth. Divide the mixture between 2 tall glasses. Top with seltzer and a scoop of frozen yogurt. Sprinkle with mint leaves.

PER FLOAT: Calories 150, protein 3 g, total fat 3 g, carbohydrates 31 g, sodium 60 mg, fiber 1 g

TINA'S TIP: Try different fruits or other berries and melons. You can also try other herbs, such as thyme, or pack a spicier punch with grated ginger.

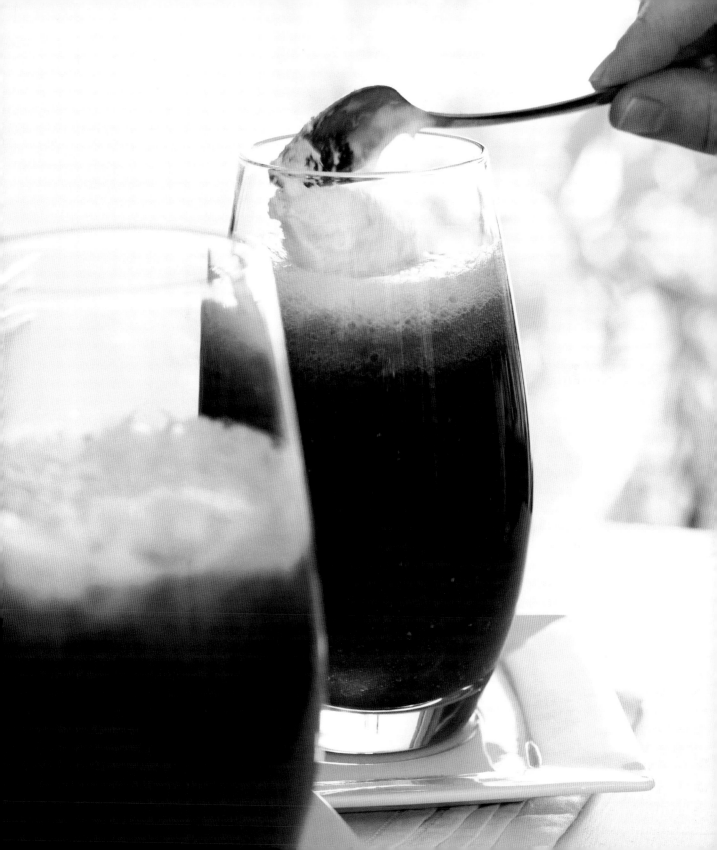

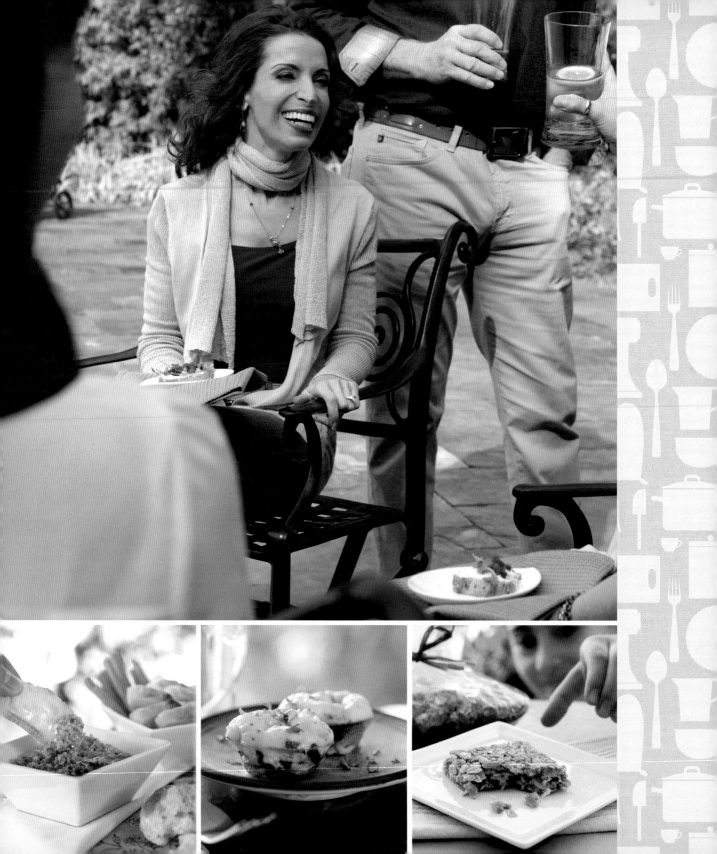

Supercharged Snacks and Nibbles

Whether it's midday or midnight, these sweet and savory munchies offer satisfaction and nutrition!

When it comes to healthy snacks, the usual suspects are downright dull. Even fruit and cheese kabobs lose their novelty. What you need are bold-flavored snacks to match today's high-octane pace. And you need snacks that satisfy, not pack on the pounds.

The secret to snacking and staying slim is limiting your snacks to 10 percent of your total calories. So, if you eat 2,000 calories each day, no more than 200 of those calories should come from snacks. Of course, growing children have greater demands for calories and nutrients, but each and every one of my snacks and nibbles will give them what they need: mega nutrition, great taste and cool new options to try.

Let's Roll!, Dynamite Egg Poppers, Naturally Nutritious Power Bars and Scoop My Salsa are just a few scrumptious snacks you'll find on the following pages. Best of all, my savory snacks can double as hors d'oeuvres!

So if you've had one too many baked chips, you're tired of low-fat dips, plain popcorn or baby carrots, and the kids really don't want any more apple wedges with peanut butter, then buckle up! This chapter is for you!

BUTTERNUT SQUASH
Mix 'n' Mash

ROASTED BUTTERNUT SQUASH MASH WITH GARLIC, WALNUTS AND OLIVE OIL

The "A" in vitamin A should stand for "amazing." It promotes healthy vision and cell development—especially important for pregnant mothers—it protects us from infection, and it may even reduce age-associated illnesses. Both animal- and plant-based foods contain vitamin A, and in this recipe, the squash is the contributor. Each tablespoon/ 14 grams of this creamy, flavor-packed dip provides nearly 70 percent of a day's worth of vitamin A and it tastes so good, you'll want to put it on everything! Of course, dips and veggies go hand in hand, but it's time to get inspired. Put a scoop of Mix 'n' Mash on your salad, spread some on your veggie burger for an extra kick of flavor or replace the mayo on your sandwich with a bit of this dip. I promise, you won't be disappointed!

YIELD: 2 cups/450 g | **TIME:** 40 minutes

---

1 butternut squash, peeled and cut into ½"/1.3 cm cubes

Salt and freshly ground pepper

1 tbsp/15 ml vegetable oil

2 tsp/10 g unsalted butter

1 clove garlic, finely chopped

¼ cup/28 g finely chopped walnuts

2 tbsp/10 g finely grated Parmigiano-Reggiano

Crostini, carrots, red peppers, radishes, etc., for dipping

Preheat oven to 400°F/200°C or gas mark 6. Place the butternut squash on a baking sheet and toss with salt, pepper and vegetable oil. Roast, turning the chunks over once or twice, until soft and golden, about 20 minutes. Place in a bowl and add the butter, garlic, walnuts and cheese. Use a heavy-duty whisk, fork or ricer to mash the squash and combine the ingredients. Taste and adjust seasoning. Serve with crostini and vegetables.

PER 1–TABLESPOON/14–GRAM SERVING: Calories 30, protein 1 g, total fat 1.5, carbohydrates 4 g, sodium 10 mg, fiber 1 g

TINA'S TIP: I always use unsalted butter when cooking. Brands differ in terms of their sodium content, and the ripeness of the produce you're using can also affect how much salt is needed. So, start with unsalted butter, and season to taste as you go.

A Star Is Born
POPCORN

PARMESAN AND ROSEMARY POPCORN

Buttered popcorn seems to be the poster child for bad food, but frankly, I like my popcorn buttered. Plain popcorn is completely uninspired, and there's no reason you have to sacrifice flavor for health. It is possible to enjoy a delicious, buttery cup of popcorn without sabotaging your diet or adding inches to your waistline or points to your cholesterol. Consider this: 1 cup/30 grams of toasted oat cereal is nearly identical to the nutrition profile of this yummy, buttered rosemary popcorn. And yes, popcorn is 100 percent whole grain. Here's my advice: make your popcorn tasty, savor every bite, and you'll be satisfied with just one serving of this salty, crunchy treat.

YIELD: 5 servings | **TIME:** 10 minutes

¼ cup/48 g popcorn kernels

5 tbsp/25 g very finely grated Parmigiano-Reggiano

2 tsp/1.5 g rosemary, very finely chopped

¼ tsp garlic powder

¼ tsp kosher salt

1 tbsp/14 g unsalted butter, melted

Using a hot air popper, pop the corn kernels. While the corn is popping, combine the cheese, rosemary, garlic powder and salt. While the popcorn is still hot, drizzle with butter and toss with the cheese mixture.

PER SERVING: Calories 90, protein 4 g, total fat 5 g, carbohydrates 8 g, sodium 220 mg, fiber 1 g

TINA'S TIP: Popcorn can take on so many different flavor profiles, so play with seasonings to create what you love! Try using curry powder and sea salt, truffle oil, cinnamon and sugar or Cajun spices. Your options are endless!

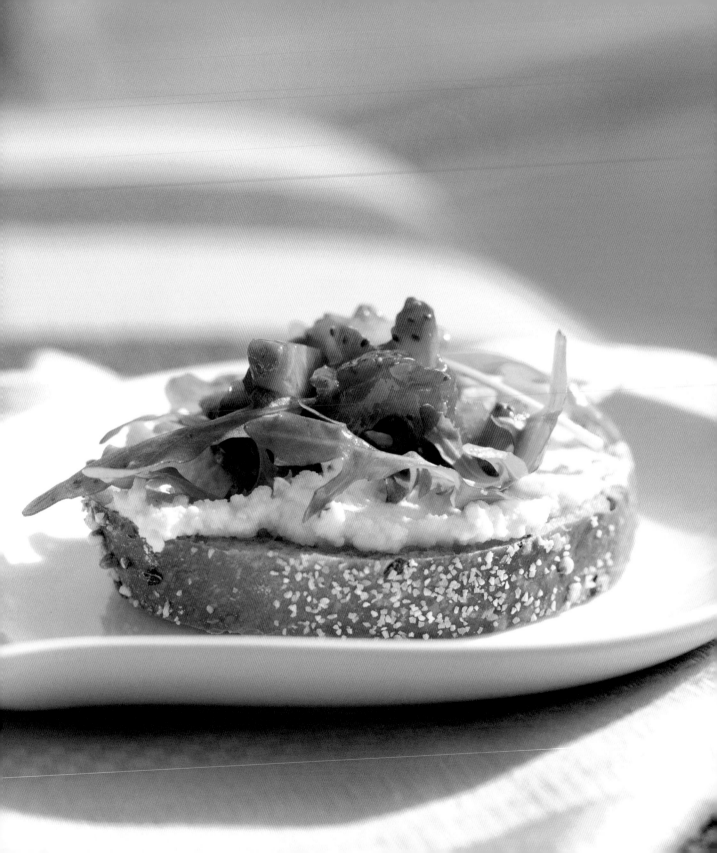

STRAWBERRIES
on a Cloud

BRUSCHETTA WITH STRAWBERRIES, RICOTTA AND ARUGULA

When you think of bruschetta (pronounced BROO-SKET-TA), odds are, you envision grilled Italian bread with chopped tomatoes on top. But this namesake dish simply means "toast." If you go to Italy, you'll find endless bruschetta varieties featuring toppings such as sausage and farmer's cheese or figs and ricotta. My version is inspired by seasonal ingredients and mouthwatering flavor combinations that make it as nutritious as it is delicious.

YIELD: 6 pieces | **TIME:** 30 minutes

1 tbsp/15 ml balsamic vinegar

½ tsp Dijon mustard

3 tbsp/45 ml olive oil

1 clove garlic, smashed

⅓ of a baguette, sliced on the diagonal into 6 slices

1 cup/170 g roughly chopped strawberries

2 tbsp/20 g finely chopped red onion

2 tsp/1.8 g basil leaves, finely sliced

Salt and freshly ground pepper

6 tbsp/94 g part-skim ricotta

2 tbsp/10 g finely grated Parmigiano-Reggiano

¼ tsp thyme leaves

¼ tsp finely grated garlic

Several grates of fresh nutmeg

1 cup/67 g arugula leaves, torn into bite-size pieces

Preheat oven to 350°F/180°C or gas mark 4. In a small bowl, combine the balsamic vinegar and Dijon mustard. Slowly whisk in the olive oil and then stir in the smashed garlic. Set aside.

Place the baguette slices on a baking tray. Bake until golden but still slightly soft in the middle, about 5 minutes. Set aside. Toasted bread can be made ahead and kept in an airtight container for 2 weeks.

In a small bowl, combine the strawberries, red onion, basil and 1 teaspoon/ 5 milliliters of vinaigrette. Sprinkle with salt and pepper.

In another small bowl, combine the ricotta, Parmigiano, thyme, grated garlic and nutmeg. Season with salt and pepper.

To assemble, place arugula in a bowl and toss with 1 teaspoon/5 milliliters vinaigrette. Divide the arugula leaves among the toasted bread. Top with ricotta mixture and finally the strawberry mixture.

PER PIECE: Calories 160, protein 5 g, total fat 9 g, carbohydrates 14 g, sodium 180 mg, fiber 1 g

TINA'S TIP: Try this with any fruit that's in season, from cherries to peaches to grapes, or a mixture of all three!

SHRIMP on a Limb

GARLIC SHRIMP AND ROASTED CHERRY TOMATO SKEWERS

Cooking fish with garlic is magical. Not only do these ingredients create mouthwatering flavors, but also both fish and garlic are effective anti-inflammatories. When combined, they interact with one another and give our bodies extra disease protection. New research shows that shrimp is a concentrated source of astaxanthin, a pigment that gives the shellfish pretty, pink color as well as the ability to fight certain cancers. With that in mind, you can feel good about serving this delicious recipe as a nutrient-rich snack or hors d'oeuvre.

YIELD: 16 skewers | **TIME:** 10 minutes

Special equipment: 16 (6"/15 cm) skewers

2 tsp/10 ml vegetable oil

16 medium shrimp, peeled and deveined

Salt and freshly ground pepper

4 cloves garlic, finely chopped

16 small red and yellow grape tomatoes

¼ cup/60 ml white wine

4 basil leaves, thinly sliced

1 tbsp/15 ml extra-virgin olive oil

Heat a sauté pan over medium heat. Add the vegetable oil to coat the bottom of the pan. Season the shrimp with salt and pepper and sauté until pink on both sides, 2 minutes per side. Add the garlic and tomatoes and cook until garlic is aromatic, about 30 seconds. Do not overcook the tomatoes or they will be too soft, making them difficult to eat. Deglaze the pan with the wine. Cook 30 seconds more. Stir in basil. Skewer 1 cherry tomato and 1 shrimp onto each of 16 skewers. Place on a serving plate and drizzle with the olive oil.

PER SKEWER: Calories 100, protein 6 g, total fat 6 g, carbohydrates 4 g, sodium 35 mg, fiber 1 g

TINA'S TIP: This also makes a nice first course served with mixed greens, or make it a main course by sautéing a few other veggies (e.g., zucchini or arugula) with the shrimp and tossing with angel hair pasta.

Let's **ROLL!**

FRESH FRUIT LEATHER

Fruit leather is like the holy grail of snacks: it's sweet, colorful, portable and fun to eat. While store-bought fruit leather is made with corn syrup, artificial colors and flavors and hydrogenated oils, my homemade version is all natural, having just three simple ingredients. Take it camping, biking or hiking, and stash in the car, your purse or a lunch bag. This homemade fruit leather will satisfy your sweet tooth without a bit of guilt!

YIELD: 12 strips | **TIME:** 55 minutes plus 3 hours baking time

1 ¼ lbs/560 g ripe fruit of your choice, roughly chopped

½ cup/100 g sugar

2 tbsp/30 ml lemon or lime juice

Preheat oven to 200°F/93°C. Place the fruit, sugar and juice in a blender, and purée until smooth. Place in a small, nonreactive saucepan and cook over low heat, stirring often, until thick, about 45 minutes. The mixture will bubble and splatter. To check that it's ready, place a spoonful of purée on a plate. Let sit for a few minutes. No water should separate out.

Line a 12 x 17-inch/30 x 43-centimeter baking tray with a silicone mat. Thinly and evenly spread the fruit purée across the baking tray in a rectangular shape. Place in the oven for about 3 hours. The purée should be slightly tacky and pull away from the silicone easily. Peel the leather off the mat and, using a ruler to guide the knife, slice into 12 even strips. Roll up and wrap in plastic wrap or place in a zip-top bag.

PER STRIP: Calories 40, protein 0 g, total fat 0 g, carbohydrates 11 g, sodium 0 g, fiber 1 g

TINA'S TIP: Instead of making strips with your fruit leather, try cutting fun shapes using cookie cutters. Also, experiment by using a combination of fruits. I like to blend together peaches, pears and strawberries, and add spices like ground coriander to give it an unexpected pop of flavor!

Flipped-Out FLAPJACKS

CURRIED VEGETABLE PANCAKES

These little curried vegetable pancakes are guaranteed to be a surprise hit. Plus, they're incredibly versatile. I love to nibble on them as a snack; made into silver dollar–size pancakes, they're a terrific hors d'oeuvre. They also work well as a simple meal when eaten alongside greens dressed with olive oil. Best of all, each pancake provides 130 percent of a day's worth of vitamin A. That's what I call tiny but mighty.

YIELD: 8 (3"/7.5 cm) pancakes | **TIME:** 30 minutes

1 small sweet potato, peeled

2 medium carrots

1 zucchini, grated

¼ tsp salt

2 scallions, finely chopped

1 tsp/2 g curry powder

1 ½ tsp/4 g grated ginger

Freshly ground pepper

3 tbsp/22 g flour

2 eggs, beaten

Vegetable oil, for sautéing

Mixed greens, for serving (optional)

Chop the sweet potato and carrots into bite-size chunks about the same size. Place the sweet potato in a pot of salted water. Bring to a boil over high heat and cook for about 15 minutes, then add the carrots and cook about 5 minutes longer, until both are soft; drain.

While they are boiling, place the zucchini in a strainer and sprinkle with salt. Set strainer in the sink to drain. After 15 minutes, rinse the zucchini and squeeze out any excess liquid. There should be ½ cup/80 g of squeezed zucchini.

Place the cooked carrots and sweet potato in the bowl of a food processor and purée until smooth. Scrape the purée into a bowl and stir in the zucchini, scallions, curry powder and ginger. Taste the mixture and season to taste with salt and pepper. Stir in the flour until just incorporated, and then stir in the eggs.

Heat a large skillet over medium heat. Brush the pan with vegetable oil. Pour ¼ cup/60 milliliters of batter onto the skillet. Pancakes will spread to approximately 3 inches/7.5 centimeters in diameter. Repeat with remaining batter. Cook the pancakes 2 to 3 minutes on the first side, or until golden brown. Flip the pancakes and cook another 2 to 3 minutes.

PER PANCAKE: Calories 60, protein 3 g, total fat 1.5 g, carbohydrates 10 g, sodium 135 mg, fiber 1 g

TINA'S TIP: These pancakes are ideal to prepare in advance. Place the cooled pancakes on a cookie sheet in the freezer. Store the frozen pancakes in a zip-top bag. To reheat, put the pancakes in a 200˚F/ 93˚C oven until warm. They're delicious as hors d'oeuvres, with a small dollop of cucumber-yogurt sauce or just plain Greek yogurt.

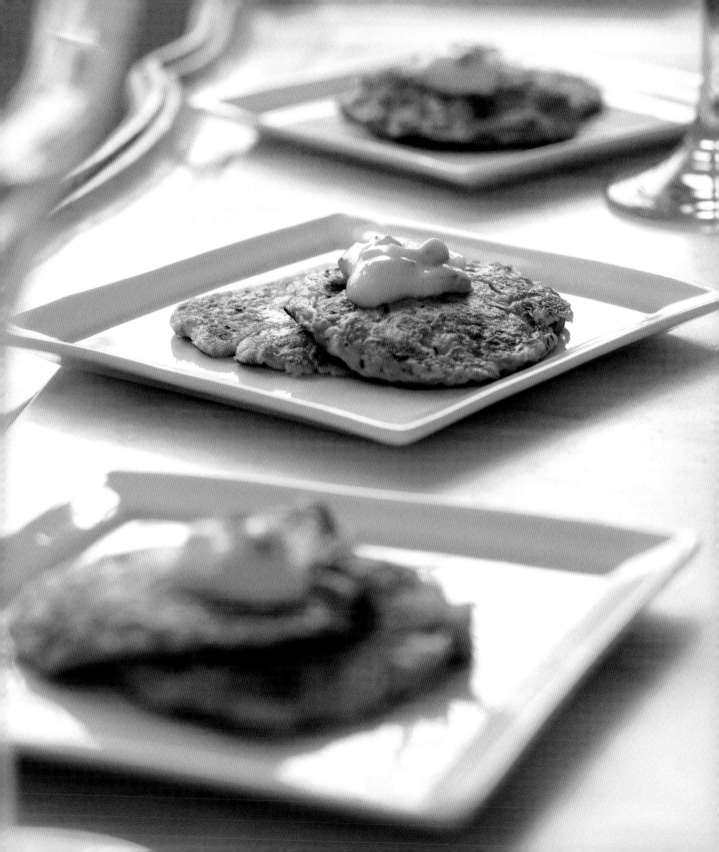

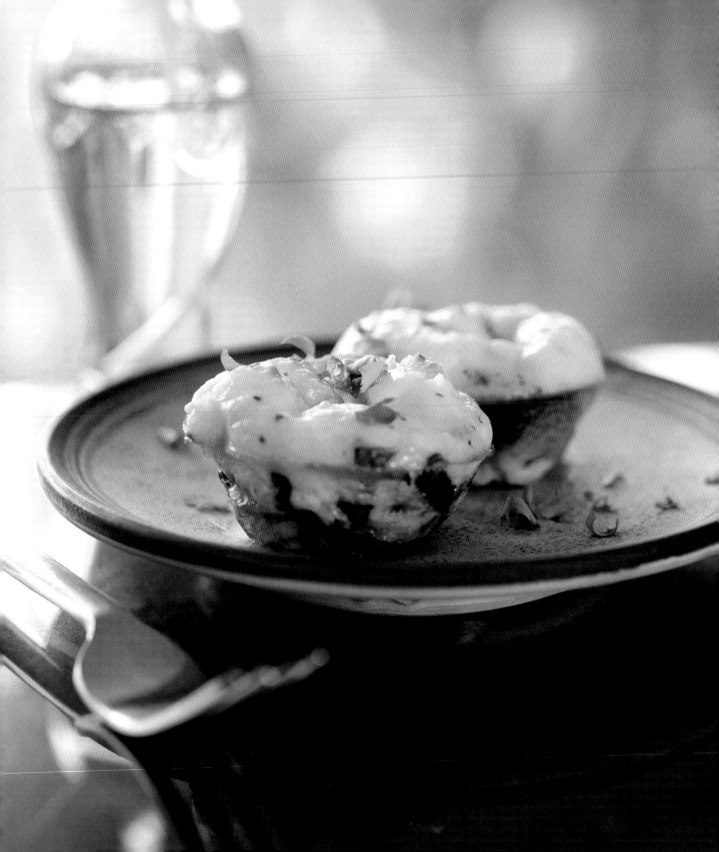

Dynamite EGG POPPERS

CRUSTLESS MINI QUICHE WITH BEET GREENS AND GOAT CHEESE

This is one of my favorite recipes in the book, and it's so simple. You can enjoy these little bites hot from the oven or cold as a snack with fresh fruit. They're a great complement to a salad (warm or at room temperature), they're a healthy hors d'oeuvre and you can make them with any greens or cheese you might have on hand. Contrary to popular belief, it's just fine to have one egg each day. Cholesterol in food isn't to blame for high blood cholesterol levels; it's saturated fat that's the culprit. And eggs are wonderfully nutritious, high in good-quality protein, vitamins, minerals and disease-fighting carotenoids.

YIELD: 24 mini quiche | **TIME:** 30 minutes

1 cup/67 g finely chopped beet greens

1 tbsp/15 ml water

Salt and freshly ground pepper

6 large eggs

½ cup/120 ml milk

¼ tsp thyme leaves

¼ cup/40 g finely chopped onion

4 oz/112 g goat cheese

1 tbsp/4 g parsley leaves, finely chopped

Preheat oven to 350°F/180°C or gas mark 4. Heat a small sauté pan over medium heat and then add the beet greens and water. Cook with a sprinkle of salt until the water has cooked away and the greens are softened, 3 to 5 minutes. Set aside.

Place the eggs, milk and thyme leaves in a bowl and whisk until the mixture is well blended; season with salt and pepper. Divide the beet greens and chopped onion among each of the 24 wells of a mini muffin tin. Top with the egg mixture. Dot the top of each mini quiche with goat cheese. Bake for 15 minutes, or until puffed and set. The quiches will fall after a few minutes—this is normal. Sprinkle with parsley and serve.

PER QUICHE: Calories 40, protein 3 g, total fat 2.5 g, carbohydrates 1 g, sodium 60 mg, fiber 0 g

TINA'S TIP: Try other flavors like sautéed mushrooms and fontina, or the classic: ham and Gruyère.

Presto **PESTO BEAN DIP**

PESTO, WHITE BEAN AND BROCCOLI DIP

You're probably familiar with pesto sauce made with basil, garlic, pine nuts and olive oil, but pesto is really a generic Italian word that refers to anything made by being pounded. Sicilians make pesto with tomatoes and, in Calabria, they make pesto with roasted red peppers. While it's fun to experiment with different variations, I don't always have time, so I use prepared pesto in this recipe. Roasting the broccoli is another little secret; it's one of the tastiest ways to cook this vegetable and requires minimal time and effort. Plus, adding broccoli means adding important phytonutrients that protect us from chronic disease and even the common cold. Broccoli is also rich in vitamin C, which fends off flu-causing viruses.

YIELD: 3 ½ cups/910 g | **TIME:** 30 minutes

1 lb/454 g broccoli florets

Salt and freshly ground pepper

2 tbsp/30 ml vegetable oil

1 (15.5 oz/434 g) can white beans, rinsed and drained

¼ cup/65 g prepared pesto sauce

Zest of ½ lemon

2 tbsp/30 ml lemon juice

1 clove garlic, finely chopped

Crostini, carrots, red peppers, radishes, etc., for dipping

Preheat oven to 400°F/200°C or gas mark 6. Place the broccoli on a baking sheet and toss with salt, pepper and vegetable oil. Roast, turning the florets over once or twice, until softened and golden, about 20 minutes. Allow to cool. Take one-quarter of the florets and finely chop them. Place the remainder in the bowl of a food processor along with the white beans, pesto sauce, lemon zest, lemon juice and garlic. Process until smooth. Place in a bowl and stir in the chopped broccoli. Adjust seasoning with salt and pepper. Serve with the crostini and vegetables.

PER 1-TABLESPOON/15-GRAM SERVING: Calories 20, protein 1 g, total fat 1 g, carbohydrates 2 g, sodium 35 mg, fiber 0 g

TINA'S TIP: Try using other beans such as chickpeas and pintos, and alter the spices such as adding cumin for a south-of-the-border flavor profile. This dip can also double as a spread on sandwiches.

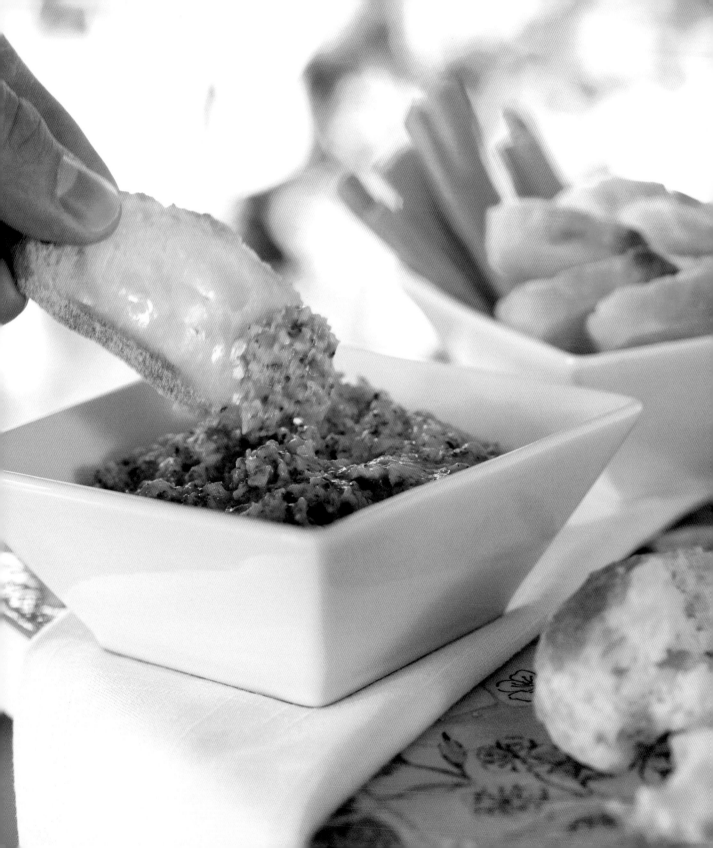

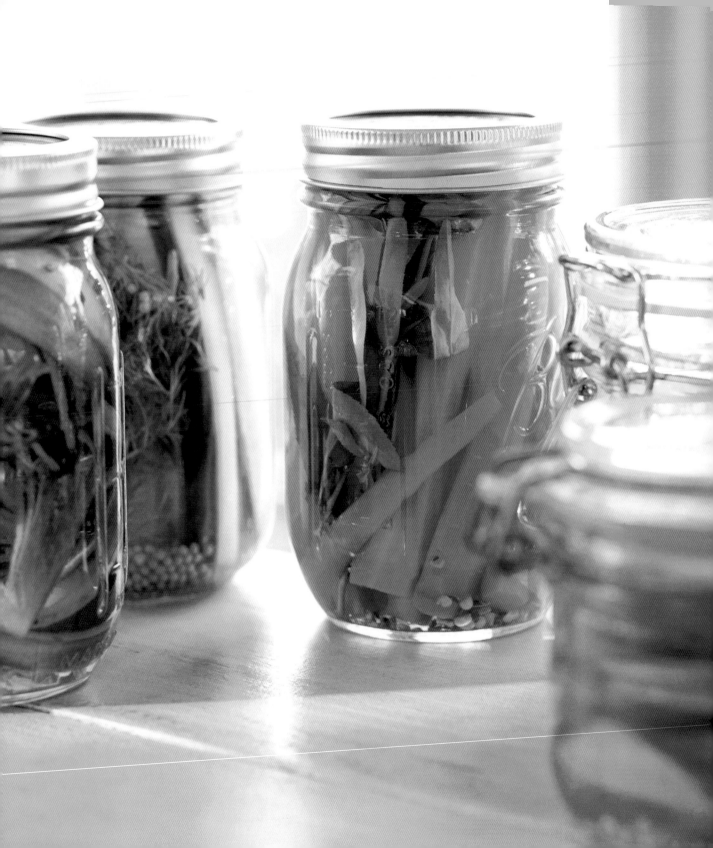

PICKLE My Fancy

QUICK PICKLED VEGETABLES

The average family throws away nearly $2,500 worth of food each year, and that waste is shameful. However, there are ways to salvage extra produce you may have on hand, before it goes bad. Pickling is a terrific solution to preserving veggies, and the method has been used effectively for thousands of years. While there are myriad different ways to pickle, my method is quick and easy and doesn't require a pressure canner. The results are yummy and gorgeous. You'll probably want to keep the jars front and center in your refrigerator; they're eye candy, not to mention mega nutritious! I also like to give these pickled vegetables as gifts, varying the produce with the season and packaging the veggies in collectible jars tied with pretty ribbon.

YIELD: 2 ½ cups/588 ml pickling brine, enough for about 4 cups/300 g cut-up vegetables
TIME: 10 minutes plus overnight pickling time

2 ½ cups/588 ml white vinegar
½ cup/100 g sugar
¼ tsp red pepper flakes
2 tsp/12 g kosher salt
1 bay leaf
1 tsp/3.7 g mustard seeds
2 tsp/3.6 g coriander seeds
2 sprigs tarragon
2 sprigs dill

Place all pickling ingredients in a nonreactive saucepan. Bring to a boil over high heat, then turn off heat; sugar should be dissolved. Place vegetables in glass jars and pour the hot pickling liquid over the vegetables. Store refrigerated.

SUGGESTED VEGETABLES:

• Kirby cucumbers, sliced into ¼-inch/6-millimeter rounds or spears
• Carrots, cut on the diagonal into ¼-inch/6-millimeter slices or spears
• Beets, cut into bite-size chunks
• Cauliflower, cut into small florets
• Celery, cut into spears
• Turnips, quartered or sliced into ¼-inch/6-millimeter rounds
• Okra
• Radishes, quartered or sliced into ¼-inch/6-millimeter rounds
• Zucchini, sliced into ¼-inch/6-millimeter rounds or spears

PER ½ CUP/40 GRAM SERVING: Calories 45, protein 1 g, total fat 0 g, carbohydrates 12 g, sodium 480 mg, fiber 1 g

TINA'S TIP: Save the pickling liquid and reuse it. Heat it again before pouring it over the vegetables.

Saucy BEEF BONBONS

MINI MEATBALLS WITH QUICK TOMATO BASIL SAUCE

I love these meatballs because they multitask. They go from snack to main dish in minutes—just add pasta! They're perfect for little mouths, but older children and adults will love them, too. Plus, they're quick and easy to make. Even the sauce can be done in a flash. Interestingly, cooking tomatoes boosts cancer-fighting power and nutritional content. Tomatoes contain lycopene, an antioxidant that gives them their gorgeous red color, and this antioxidant increases with heat, making lycopene the most efficient oxygen quencher we know of. What does that mean? It means that lycopene is like Pac-Man when it comes to devouring free radicals, gobbling up the bad guys to keep you healthy!

YIELD: 18 meatballs | **TIME:** 35 minutes

FOR THE MEATBALLS:

1 lb/455 g ground beef

6 tbsp/42 g breadcrumbs

2 cloves garlic, finely chopped

1 small onion, finely chopped

Pinch of ground nutmeg

¼ cup/15 g parsley, finely chopped

1 egg

Salt and freshly ground pepper

FOR THE SAUCE:

2 tbsp/30 ml vegetable oil

½ cup/80 g finely chopped onion

4 cloves garlic, finely chopped

1 ½ tsp/1.2 g thyme leaves

1 tbsp/16 g tomato paste

1 (28 oz/784 g) can crushed tomatoes

½ cup/120 ml water

4 basil leaves, finely sliced

½ oz/14 g Parmigiano-Reggiano

To make the meatballs, place beef, breadcrumbs, garlic, onion, nutmeg, parsley and egg in medium bowl. Season with salt and pepper. Mix well to incorporate all ingredients. Divide the mixture into 18 mini meatballs, rolling them in the palms of your hands. To firm up the meat, refrigerate the meatballs while making the sauce.

To make the sauce, place a large saucepan over medium heat. Add the vegetable oil and sauté the onion until golden, 2 minutes. Add the garlic and thyme and cook until aromatic, another 30 seconds. Add the tomato paste and stir to allow the tomato paste to caramelize, about 1 minute. Add the canned tomatoes and water, and simmer the sauce, covered, for 10 minutes.

Place the meatballs in the sauce. Cover the saucepan and simmer for 10 minutes. Carefully shake the pan to turn the meatballs, or gently rotate them with a spoon, to ensure they get covered with sauce. Continue to simmer for an additional 5 to 10 minutes, or until the meatballs are cooked through. Sprinkle generously with freshly chopped basil and cheese.

PER MEATBALL: Calories 90, protein 5 g, total fat 7 g, carbohydrates 2 g, sodium 75 mg, fiber 0 g

PER ¼ CUP/60 MILLILITERS SAUCE: Calories 35, protein 1 g, total fat 2 g, carbohydrates 0 g, sodium 130 mg, fiber 1 g

TINA'S TIP: The meatballs and sauce can last 5 days in the refrigerator. You can serve them over pasta, in a toasted hero sandwich with melted provolone or as a hearty snack. To freeze, place the cooked meatballs and sauce into separate containers. They will last up to 1 month.

Irresistible
ALMOND-GARLIC DIP

WHIPPED SWEET POTATOES WITH GARLIC, OLIVE OIL AND ALMONDS

When I tire of hummus and want a change, I make this recipe. Skordalia is a thick and creamy purée of Greek origin and it's made by blending potatoes with garlic, olive oil, crushed walnuts and almonds. I whip up my own version with sweet potatoes, and the secret to making this dip extra healthy is to boil the sweet potatoes! Research shows that boiling sweet potatoes, instead of roasting or baking them, makes the spud more effective at stabilizing blood sugar. Boiled sweet potatoes have also been shown to increase blood levels of vitamin A in children. Just 1 tablespoon/14 grams of my skordalia provides 40 percent of a day's worth of vitamin A and a whole lot of flavor!

YIELD: 4 cups/900 g | **TIME:** 30 minutes

3 medium sweet potatoes, peeled

5 cloves garlic, smashed

1 cup/110 g slivered almonds, toasted

5 tbsp/75 ml lemon juice

¼ cup/60 ml extra-virgin olive oil

Salt and freshly ground pepper

Toasted pita bread cut into triangles, for dipping

Cut the sweet potatoes into large chunks and place in a pot of salted water. Boil until soft, about 15 minutes, and drain.

In the bowl of a food processor, add the garlic, almonds, lemon juice and olive oil. Purée until fairly smooth. Add the sweet potatoes, and pulse, scraping down the sides of the bowl from time to time, until the potatoes have completely broken down. Add salt and pepper to taste. Serve with pita bread.

PER 1-TABLESPOON/14-GRAM SERVING: Calories 30, protein 1 g, total fat 2 g, carbohydrates 3 g, sodium 10 mg, fiber 1 g

TINA'S TIP: When peeling several cloves of garlic, the skins become very sticky. To avoid this, smash the cloves with the side of a chef's knife and then place them in a small bowl of cool water. The skins will slip right off!

CHOCOLATE PEANUT BUTTER Power Bites

CHUNKY PEANUT BUTTER BALLS WITH COCOA AND DRIED CHERRIES

There are times when I want a sweet treat, but I only need a little taste of something to be satisfied. The answer? These tiny, yummy, chewy bites of peanut butter, cocoa and dried cherries! They're the perfect, guilt-free snack that you can enjoy without packing on pounds. They can be made in just minutes, too. The dough is a bit sticky, but that makes it ideal for the coconut to adhere. While you're at it, toast extra coconut to have on hand. I keep toasted coconut in a glass jar in my pantry, and toss it into oatmeal and smoothies and sprinkle it on frozen yogurt. Otherwise, keep these little bites refrigerated, and they'll last for days.

YIELD: 14 pieces | **TIME:** 10 minutes

2 tbsp/32 g chunky peanut butter

1 tbsp/8 g unsweetened cocoa powder

3 tbsp/45 ml honey

2 tbsp/10 g quick cooking oats

3 tbsp/15 g toasted unsweetened coconut, plus additional for rolling

¼ cup/30 g dried cherries, roughly chopped

Place all ingredients in a bowl and use a wooden spoon or rubber spatula to combine well. Divide into 14 pieces and roll into balls, then press into remaining coconut. Refrigerate.

PER PIECE: Calories 45, protein 1 g, total fat 2 g, carbohydrates 7 g, sodium 10 mg, fiber 1 g

TINA'S TIP: Try using other nut butters like almond or cashew along with other dried fruit. For an adult twist, try adding spices like coriander, cumin and even cayenne.

Scoop MY SALSA

GREEK SALAD SALSA

This salsa has all the healthy ingredients and flavors of a Greek salad, but in scoopable form! How fun is that? Enjoy this as a dip, pita filling or salad topping. For extra flavor, I toss in a bit of mint, which contains essential minerals such as manganese, copper, iron, potassium and calcium. Although mint is eaten in small quantities, its nutrients are still beneficial to health.

YIELD: 4 cups/900 g | **TIME:** 20 minutes

3 plum tomatoes, seeded and finely chopped

1 cup/120 g finely chopped cucumber

¾ cup/112 g crumbled feta cheese

1 small red onion, finely chopped

10 mint leaves, chopped

1 tsp/1.3 g fresh oregano

½ cup/50 g , pitted and finely chopped kalamata olives or other oil-cured black olives

2 tbsp/30 ml extra-virgin olive oil

1 tbsp/15 ml red wine vinegar

Salt and freshly ground pepper

Toasted pita triangles, for serving

Combine all ingredients except pita. Add salt and pepper to taste. Serve with pita bread.

PER 1-TABLESPOON/14-GRAM SERVING: Calories 80, protein 4 g, total fat 6 g, carbohydrates 3 g, sodium 270 mg, fiber 1 g

TINA'S TIP: When seeding a tomato, don't throw the seeds away! Add them to the blender when you make vinaigrette or a smoothie. It will add a fresh flavor and even more nutrition.

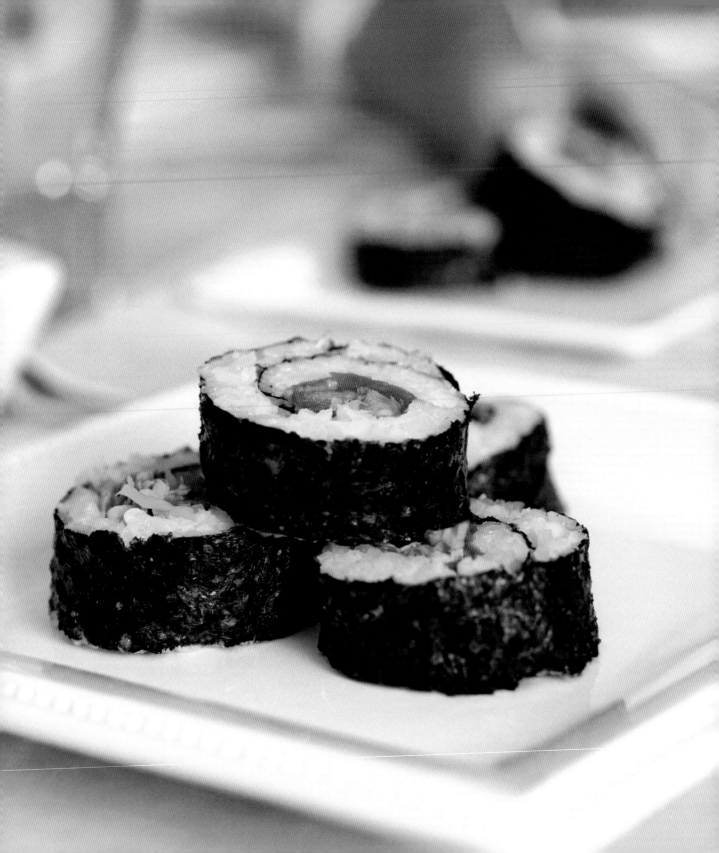

ROLL Model

TURKEY BACON SUSHI ROLLS

These sushi rolls make the perfect, balanced snack. They have a little bit of protein, energy-boosting carbohydrates and some satiating fat; they're easy to hold, are fun to eat, and they taste great, too! I've incorporated quinoa into the rice for a protein boost, but it does make the rice a little less sticky, so be sure to roll the sushi as tightly as possible. While a bamboo mat can be used to roll the sushi, a square of heavy-duty foil can be used as a substitute. Last year, I made these sushi rolls for a Super Bowl party appetizer, and they were a huge hit with young and old alike!

YIELD: 5 sushi rolls, 35 pieces | **TIME:** 45 minutes

1 cup/195 g sushi rice

⅓ cup/58 g quinoa

1 ¾ cups/420 ml water

2 ½ tbsp/37.5 seasoned rice vinegar

12 slices turkey bacon

1 (6 oz/170 g) package toasted nori sheets

1 large tomato, thinly sliced

1 ½ cups/100 g shredded romaine lettuce

Reduced-sodium soy sauce, for serving

Wasabi, for serving

Pickled ginger, for serving

Preheat oven to 375°F/190°C or gas mark 5. In a medium stockpot, add sushi rice, quinoa and water. Bring to a boil over high heat. Cover, reduce heat to low, and let mixture cook 20 minutes. Remove from heat, and let rice sit 10 additional minutes. Stir rice vinegar into rice before using. Meanwhile, layer turkey bacon onto a baking sheet. Bake according to package directions, about 8 to 12 minutes. Remove from oven, and let cool.

To assemble the sushi, line up all the ingredients and cover the bamboo rolling mat with plastic wrap. Place 1 sheet of nori on top of a rolling mat, shiny-side-down. Lightly spread about ¾ cup/180 milliliters rice mixture in an even layer on nori. Layer the strip of nori closest to you with 1 ½ to 2 pieces bacon, 3 slices of tomatoes and shredded lettuce. Using your fingers to keep the filling in place, roll the mat (and nori) into a cylinder shape, using the mat to shape the entire roll. Squeeze tightly. Remove the mat, and continue to roll sushi. Using a sharp knife, cut roll into 7 pieces, and place on a platter. Repeat process until all the rice is used, which will make approximately 5 rolls. Serve with soy sauce, wasabi and pickled ginger.

PER PIECE: Calories 60, protein 3 g, total fat 2 g, carbohydrates 8 g, sodium 110 mg, fiber 3 g

TINA'S TIP: Different varieties of lettuce can be used, instead of romaine. Also, avocado slices can be incorporated into these sushi rolls along with a bit of light mayonnaise.

Naturally Nutritious
POWER BARS

APRICOT-COCONUT GRANOLA BARS

Most granola bars are really just candy bars in disguise. My apricot-coconut granola bars are a yummy alternative to what you find on the shelf. Apricots are a source of vitamins A and C, and the minerals calcium, potassium and iron. Their powerful antioxidants are protective against age-related macular degeneration. Coconuts contain lauric acid, which is antiviral and antibacterial and boosts immunity. These snacks travel beautifully, whether in a lunch bag or handbag, and they'll last up to 5 days in a tightly sealed container. Use the crumbles in a yogurt parfait, and nothing will go to waste!

YIELD: 20 squares | **TIME:** 50 minutes plus 5 to 6 hours cooling time

2 cups/160 g old-fashioned rolled oats

1 ¼ cups/106 g shredded unsweetened coconut

¾ cup/109 g unsalted sunflower seeds or unsalted peanuts

1 cup/130 g dried apricots, roughly chopped

½ cup/60 g vanilla protein powder

¼ tsp salt

¼ cup/60 g brown sugar, packed

¾ cup/180 ml maple syrup

2 tbsp/28 g unsalted butter, cut into pieces

Preheat oven to 325°F/170°C or gas mark 3. Line a rimmed baking sheet with foil or parchment paper. Add oats and coconut and bake until toasted, about 15 to 20 minutes, stirring mixture every 5 minutes. Remove from oven, and reserve. Meanwhile, place sunflower seeds or nuts and dried apricots into the bowl of a food processor. Pulse mixture for 30 seconds to 1 minute, until apricots and seeds are tiny bits without being completely puréed.

Coat a 9 x 12-inch/23 x 30-centimeter baking dish very lightly with cooking spray. Set aside. In a large bowl, add apricot mixture, protein powder, salt and reserved oat-coconut mixture. In a small stockpot, add brown sugar, maple syrup and butter. Stir mixture over medium-high heat until butter is melted. Remove from heat, and carefully pour into oat mixture. Stir to combine until entire mixture is coated. Transfer mixture into prepared baking dish. Using your hands or a spatula, firmly press down on oat mixture, packing it into the dish. Bake for 20 minutes for a chewier granola bar, 25 minutes for a crunchier one. Granola mixture will be golden around the edges of the pan. Remove from oven. Using a spatula, firmly press down on mixture again. Cover and let sit at room temperature for at least 5 to 6 hours. Using a serrated knife, cut the granola bars into 20 squares. Store in an airtight container.

PER SQUARE: Calories 180, protein 4 g, total fat 7 g, carbohydrates 24 g, sodium 35 mg, fiber 3 g

TINA'S TIP: This makes such a pretty gift! You can wrap the bars individually or in batches. And, these bars can be frozen, so you can bake now and wrap later!

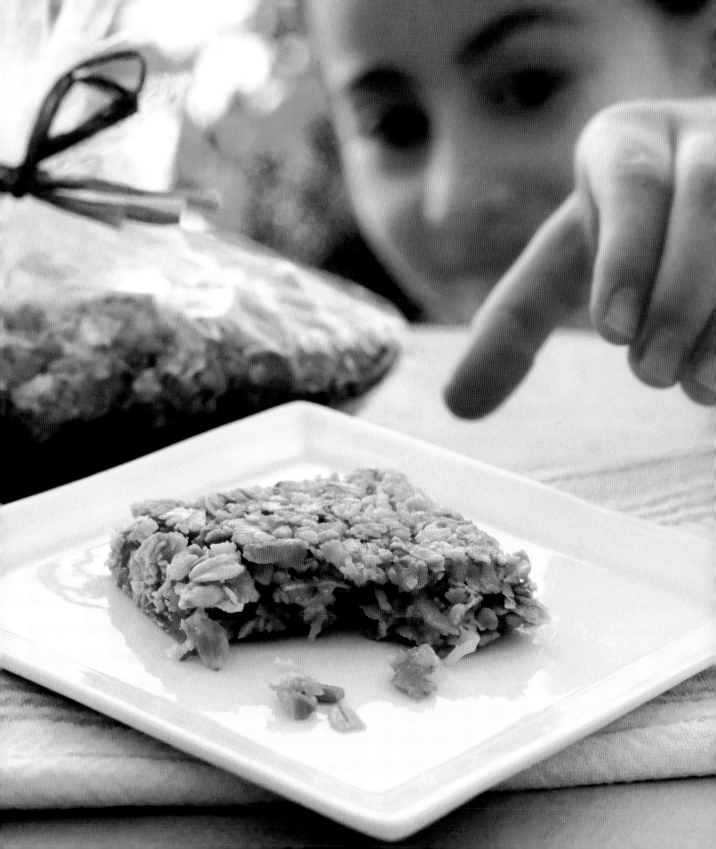

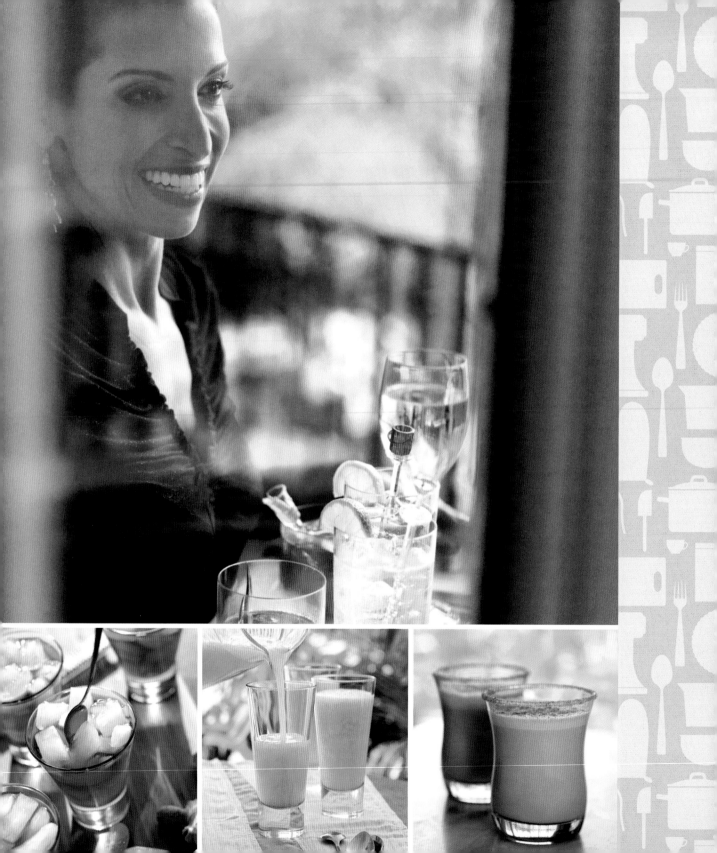

Luscious Libations

Perk up your days and nights with healthy coffees, teas and skinny cocktails!

Most family cookbooks never include drinks, and I often wonder why. Women consume 25 percent of their calories from beverages, and American women have five alcoholic beverages each week, with vodka being their favorite choice in cocktails.

Let's face it: a well-chosen beverage—alcoholic or not—can make a meal that much more delicious and enjoyable. Imagine teatime without tea. Those little finger sandwiches would not be complete. Cookies without milk? Santa would strike. A good drink is essential to satisfaction, and beverages can be a source of nutrition, as well.

Coffee gets a bum rap, but new research shows it can be good for you, improving stamina before a workout, enhancing concentration and even protecting you from Alzheimer's disease. Tea helps protect us from cardiovascular disease and fights free radicals. Green tea, in particular, has been found to improve bone density and strength.

Today, alcohol's stigma endures even though scientific evidence shows moderate drinkers may live longer and be healthier than those who don't drink at all. So, what should you be drinking? There's good news for beer, wine and spirit lovers. Major research shows each type of alcohol equally paves a route to health, which means it's not what you drink, but how much you drink that's important.

A drink a day can keep the doctor at bay, so clink to health when you try this yummy collection of liquid bliss! Salute!

South-of-the-Border
SOOTHER

HOT SPICED COCOA

This scrumptious hot cocoa has delicate notes of cinnamon and a rich chocolate taste and looks so pretty when garnished with a cinnamon stick. Consuming just a ½ teaspoon of cinnamon daily has the power to lower your LDL cholesterol, and it works to stabilize blood pressure, fight bacteria and boost cognition. Best of all, cinnamon is downright comforting, making this the perfect beverage to help you de-stress!

YIELD: 1 serving | **TIME:** 5 minutes

½ tsp cocoa, unsweetened

Dash of cinnamon

1 tsp/5 ml hot water

½ cup/120 ml hot coffee

¼ cup/60 ml nonfat or low-fat milk

Cinnamon stick or ground cinnamon, for garnish

Combine the cocoa powder, cinnamon and hot water in the bottom of a mug. Pour coffee over the cocoa mixture. Steam the milk on a cappuccino machine, with a milk frother, or just heat milk to simmer, and then pour into mug. Garnish with cinnamon stick or a dash of ground cinnamon.

PER SERVING: Calories 30, protein 2 g, total fat 0 g, carbohydrates 5 g, sodium 35 mg, fiber 1 g

TINA'S TIP: To make this for a crowd, sprinkle the cinnamon on the coffee in the coffee filter basket and brew as usual.

Razzle Dazzle
BERRY MOCHA

ICED RASPBERRY MOCHA

You probably wouldn't think of tossing raspberries into your iced coffee, but the combination is incredible! This iced mocha has a bright berry flavor that's not sweet yet satisfying. It also packs 25 percent of your daily need for calcium and one-third of a day's worth of vitamin C into each serving. What's more, you're doing something good for your heart with each sip: raspberries are linked to lower heart disease risk and new research shows that eating berries at a very early age may reduce a woman's risk of heart attack later in life—a profound finding because heart disease is the number one killer of women.

YIELD: 1 serving | **TIME:** 5 minutes

6 oz/180 ml coffee, chilled
½ cup/125 g raspberries, frozen
1 tsp/4 g sugar
1 tsp/2 g cocoa, unsweetened
½ cup/120 ml nonfat milk, frozen
(4 cubes, see tip)

Combine all ingredients in a blender and purée until smooth. Pour into serving glass. Enjoy your beverage!

PER SERVING: Calories 110, protein 6 g, total fat 0.5 g, carbohydrates 20 g, sodium 70 mg, fiber 2 g

TINA'S TIP: Freeze milk in ice cube trays, so it's ready for the blender.

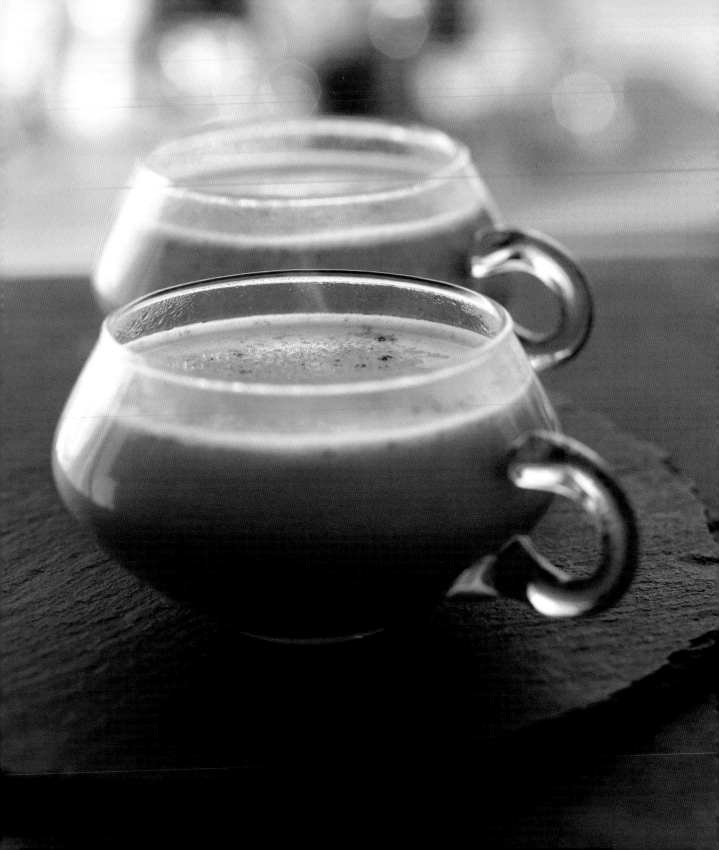

SPICE Is Nice!

CREAMY PUMPKIN COFFEE

Canned pumpkin is a great source of vitamins A and C, and it's available year-round, when winter squash can't be found. I use canned pumpkin all the time because it's nutrient-rich and low in fat and calories. Just make sure you buy 100 percent pure pumpkin and not pumpkin pie filling! This delicious, creamy pumpkin drink supplies 90 percent of your daily vitamin A needs and 25 percent of your daily calcium requirements.

YIELD: 1 serving | **TIME:** 5 minutes

¾ cup/180 ml low-fat milk

2 tsp/8 g sugar, brown or white

2 tbsp/30 g pumpkin purée

¼ tsp vanilla extract

2 dashes of nutmeg

Dash of cinnamon

Pinch of ground ginger

½ cup/120 ml hot coffee

Combine the milk, sugar, pumpkin purée, vanilla, nutmeg, cinnamon and ginger in a blender and blend on high speed to purée, creating a frothy consistency. Pour into a saucepan and heat until hot but do not boil. Pour hot coffee into mug and top with hot spiced milk.

PER SERVING: Calories 120, protein 7 g, total fat 2 g, carbohydrates 20 g, sodium 85 mg, fiber 1 g

TINA'S TIP: This coffee is also delicious iced. Freeze the leftover pumpkin and use it in smoothies, pumpkin bread or pumpkin muffins.

Creamy Dreamy
ORANGE TEA

ORANGE AND CREAM ICED TEA

You've probably never heard of hesperidin, but it's a powerful antioxidant that's found in orange peels. Most people love oranges, but they don't think about the peel when they toss it after juicing. Next time, save the peel and zest it. Hesperidin can lower blood pressure and regulate cholesterol levels, in addition to being an effective anti-inflammatory. Additionally, orange peels can add brightness and be a delicious finishing touch! This recipe utilizes both orange juice and orange zest to create a drink that's part iced tea, part creamsicle. Plus, it provides 50 percent of a day's worth of immune-boosting vitamin C.

YIELD: 1 serving | **TIME:** 10 minutes

2 orange pekoe tea bags (or any other type of black tea)

1 cup/235 ml boiling water

¾ tsp orange zest

¼ cup/60 ml freshly squeezed orange juice

2 tsp/10 ml honey

3 tbsp/45 ml whole milk

3 or 4 ice cubes

Add the tea bags to the boiling water, letting the tea steep for 5 minutes. Remove tea bags and discard them. Add tea to a blender, along with orange zest, orange juice, honey, milk and ice cubes. Whirl ingredients in blender until ice has dissolved, about 1 to 2 minutes. Serve immediately.

PER SERVING: Calories 100, protein 2 g, total fat 1.5 g, carbohydrates 22 g, sodium 85 mg, fiber 0 g

TINA'S TIP: Any type of tea can be used, including decaffeinated or green tea. As for the orange zest, try it in risotto, marinades or salad dressing.

Earl Grey **PEAR LATTE**

PEAR-HONEY TEA

I love pears, and when it comes to fruit, they seem to be unsung heroes. Perhaps it's their modest shape or earthy colors, but they don't grace magazine food pages like ruby-red raspberries or plump, sultry blackberries. It's time pears got their due! New research shows that among all fruits and vegetables, pears demonstrate the most consistent ability to lower the risk of type 2 diabetes. They also have antioxidant and anticancer properties and are a good source of fiber, potassium and vitamins A and C. In this tea, they play a starring role, imparting a sweet taste and satisfying texture.

YIELD: 1 serving | **TIME:** 10 minutes

½ cup/120 ml prepared Earl Grey tea

2 oz/56 g peeled and diced ripe pear

1 tsp/5 ml honey

Dash of cinnamon

½ cup/120 ml nonfat milk

Place Earl Grey tea, diced pear, honey and cinnamon in a saucepan and cook until softened, 5 minutes. Pour into a blender and purée until smooth. Take care when blending hot liquids. Pour into mug. Steam the milk on a cappuccino machine, with a milk frother or just heat milk to simmer and pour into mug.

PER SERVING: Calories 100, protein 4 g, total fat 0 g, carbohydrates 21 g, sodium 65 mg, fiber 4 g

TINA'S TIP: Experiment with different pear varieties. I like Comice pears, which have an exceptionally soft, sweet flesh. Red Anjou, Bosc and Seckel pears will also work well.

HIBISCUS-GINGER
Refresher

ICED GREEN TEA WITH MANGO AND LIME

Tea is an age-old elixir, and new studies show that tea may help enhance immunity, lower bad cholesterol levels and even reduce the risk of cancer. Some science even shows that tea is an effective antimicrobial. To get the maximum health benefits from this delicious drink, steep your tea for 3 minutes, then prepare the recipe as written.

YIELD: 1 serving | **TIME:** 5 minutes

¼ cup/60 ml mango nectar

½ cup/120 ml prepared hibiscus tea, chilled

½ tsp grated ginger

Ice cubes

Lime wedge, for garnish

Stir together the mango nectar, tea and ginger. Pour into a highball glass packed with ice. Give it one good stir and serve garnished with a lime wedge.

PER SERVING: Calories 30, protein 0 g, total fat 0 g, carbohydrates 7 g, sodium 0 mg, fiber 0 mg

TINA'S TIP: Rim the glass with lime for added flavor.

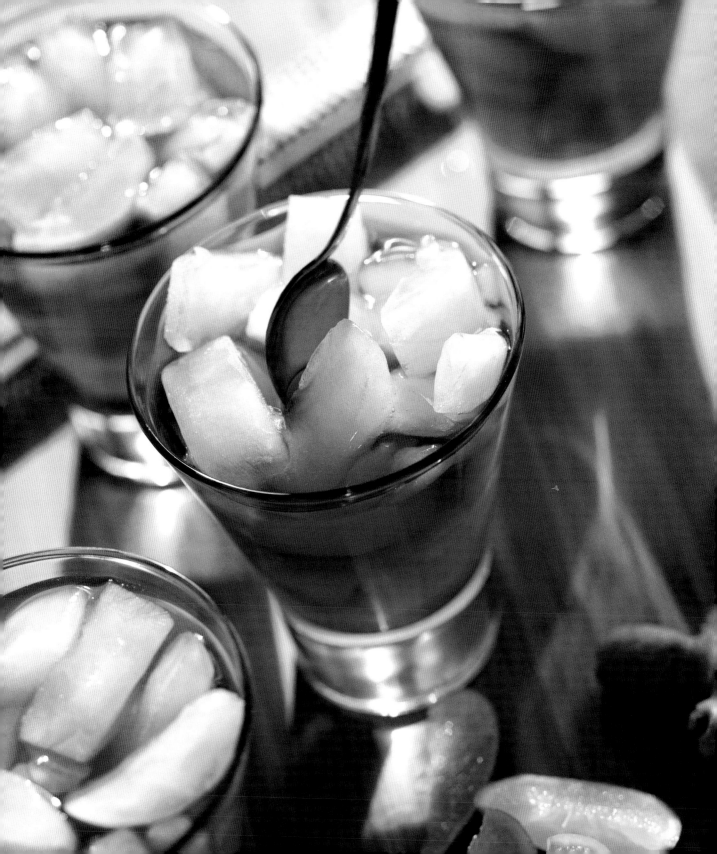

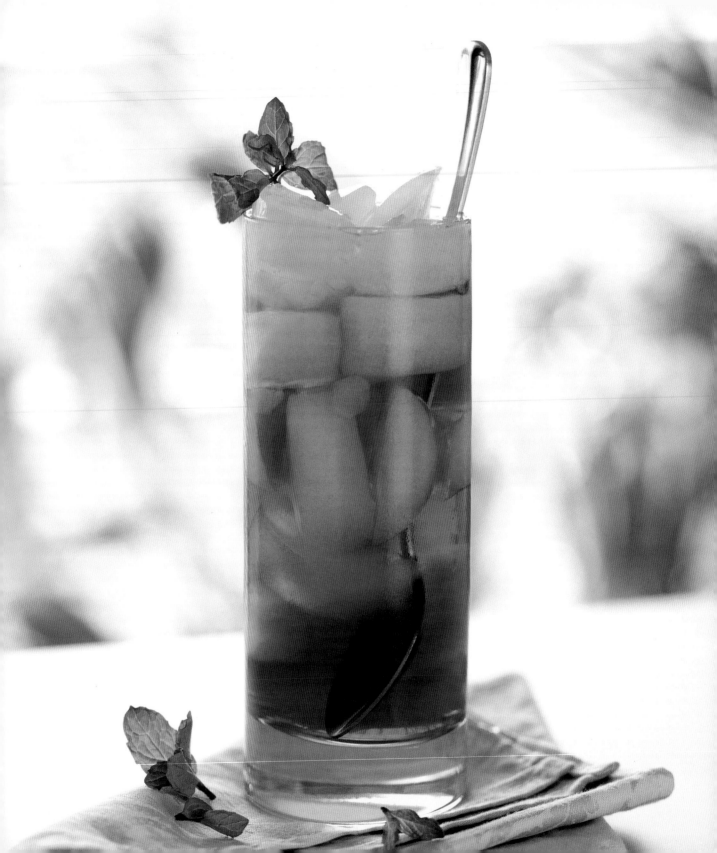

"MIN-TEA" Energizer

HONEY-MINT GREEN TEA

We're all familiar with mint's refreshing taste, but mint has extraordinary medicinal properties, from soothing an upset tummy and relieving asthma to fighting germs and promoting digestion. Honey, a powerful antioxidant, also has antiviral and antibacterial properties and promotes digestive health. Combined, these ingredients make a cool, crisp and delicate beverage—a wonderful afternoon pick-me-up or a memorable drink for a luncheon or shower!

YIELD: 1 serving | **TIME:** 5 minutes

1 bag green tea

¾ cup/180 ml water

5 fresh mint leaves or 1 bag mint tea

2 tsp/10 ml honey

Ice cubes

Club soda (optional)

1 sprig mint, for garnish

Brew green tea in the water with the mint leaves or mint tea bag and honey. Steep according to taste. Cool and strain into a highball packed with ice. Top with club soda, if desired, and give it one good stir. Garnish with mint sprig.

PER SERVING: Calories 45, protein 0 g, total fat 0 g, carbohydrates 11 g, sodium 5 mg, fiber 0 g

Orange Vodka
SNOWBALL

VODKA-SPIKED COFFEE WITH ORANGE LIQUEUR AND FROZEN YOGURT

Alcohol has a stigma that endures, even though scientific findings show that light to moderate drinking can have health benefits. Additionally, we know alcohol has calories, but drinking alcohol doesn't lead to weight gain in and of itself. So, go ahead and indulge in this guilt-free treat after a long day and the kids have gone to bed. I promise it will be a memorable nightcap!

YIELD: 1 serving | **TIME:** 5 minutes

½ cup/120 g nonfat coffee-flavored frozen yogurt

¼ cup/60 ml chilled, brewed coffee

1 tbsp/15 ml vodka

1 tbsp/15 ml orange-flavored liqueur

Orange slice, for garnish

Pour all ingredients except orange slice into a blender. Mix on high for 30 seconds, or until drink is smooth and creamy. Pour into a chilled glass and garnish with orange slice.

PER SERVING: Calories 190, protein 3 g, total fat 5 g, carbohydrates 22 g, sodium 70 mg, fiber 0 g

TINA'S TIP: To enhance drink presentation, rim the glass with cinnamon- sugar. To do so, run an orange wedge around the rim. Next, invert the glass and dip it into a plate of superfine sugar mixed with cinnamon. Garnish with orange slice, as directed above.

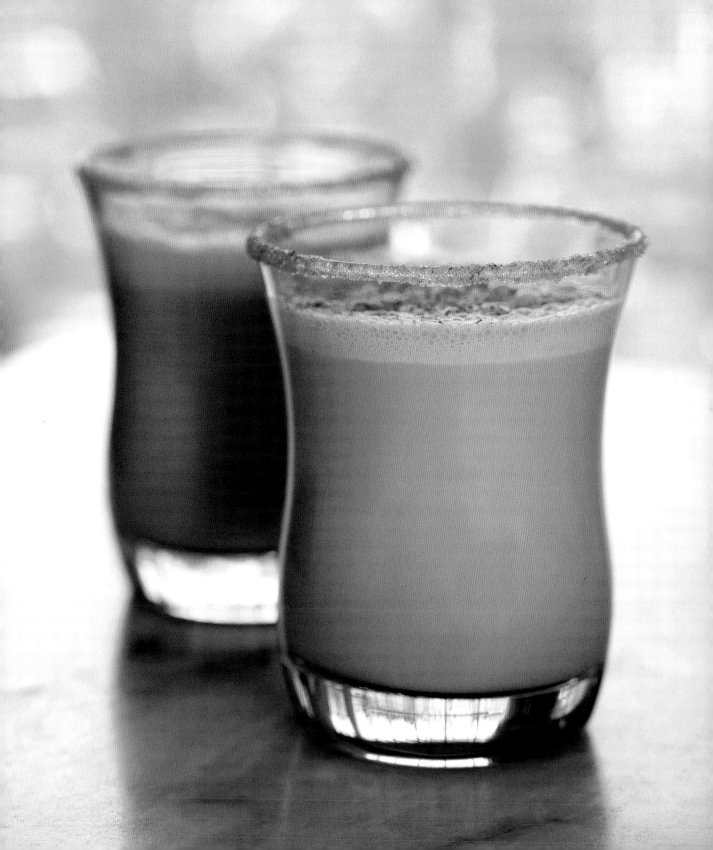

Blueberry CASSIS FIZZ

LIGHT VODKA CRANBERRY WITH CASSIS AND BLUEBERRIES

Great finger foods (like those found in this book!) can make the perfect cocktail even better, and when that cocktail is "skinny," it's a marriage made in heaven! This vodka drink is perfect for the over-twenty-one crowd, and it's especially appealing because it doesn't contain any artificial ingredients. The fizziness from the sparkling wine adds a welcoming element, and the blueberries provide a nice addition of good-for-you antioxidants!

YIELD: 1 serving | **TIME:** 5 minutes

6 blueberries

1 tbsp/15 ml cassis

2 tbsp/30 ml vodka

2 tbsp/30 ml light cranberry juice

Ice cubes

6 tbsp/90 ml rosé sparkling wine, cold

Lemon twist, for garnish

3 blueberries on a toothpick, for garnish

Place blueberries, cassis, vodka and cranberry juice into a rocks glass. Muddle the berries well. Add ice and pour in the sparkling wine. Give a quick stir and garnish with the lemon twist and blueberries on a toothpick.

PER SERVING: Calories 180, protein 0 g, total fat 0 g, carbohydrates 10 g, sodium 5 mg, fiber 0 g

TINA'S TIP: Blackberries can be substituted for the blueberries, and they make a beautiful garnish!

Ginger ROGERS

GINGER MARTINI

A shaker packed with ice, a beautiful glass and a few quality ingredients are the essence of a great martini, and when it's time for the adults to get together, I love nothing more than serving a memorable one. Recent scientific evidence shows that moderate drinkers live longer and are healthier than those who don't drink at all, so why not indulge? Not that you'll go overboard with this drink! It's crisp, light and a ginger lover's paradise. Aromatic and spicy, ginger has been shown to help alleviate everything from symptoms of the common cold to inflammation and even boost immunity. Cheers!

YIELD: 1 serving | **TIME:** 5 minutes

¼ cup/60 ml peach nectar

1 tbsp/15 ml fresh lime juice

¼ tsp grated fresh ginger

3 tbsp/45 ml gin

1 peach slice, for garnish

Place all the ingredients except the garnish in a cocktail shaker packed with ice. Shake well and strain into a martini glass. Garnish with the peach slice.

PER SERVING: Calories 140, protein 0 g, total fat 0 g, carbohydrates 11 g, sodium 0 mg, fiber 1 g

TINA'S TIP: The smaller the pieces of ginger, the more they'll incorporate into the drink. So, grate the ginger with a zester, such as a Microplane, for best results. Don't have one? Go get one because it's the best kitchen tool you can have! It's designed to extract the finest flavor from your food in just the perfect size. I also use mine when working with hard cheese, onions and citrus fruit.

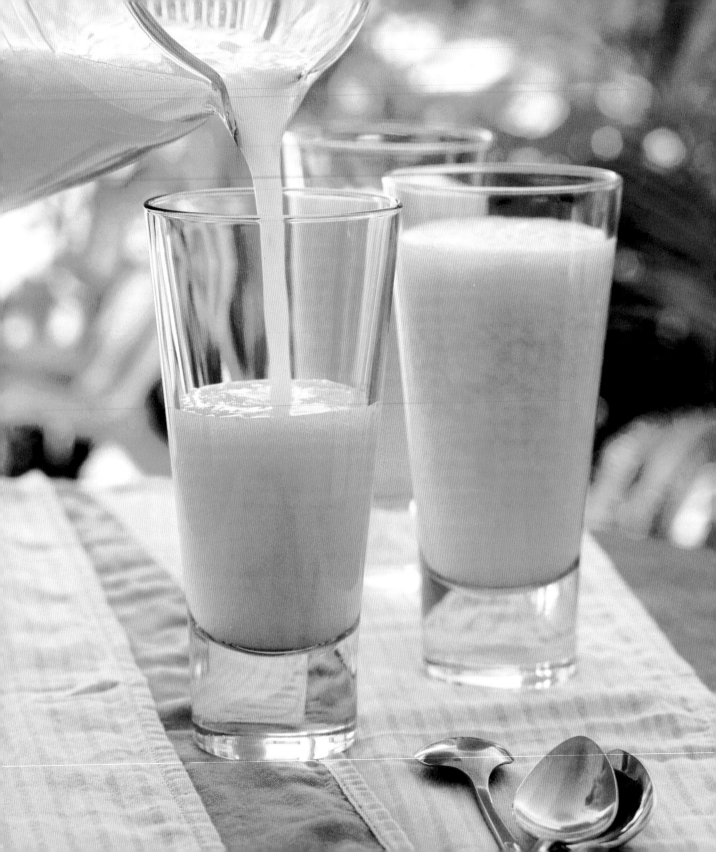

Honolulu **BREEZE**

SKINNY RUM-KISSED BANANA AND PINEAPPLE HIGHBALL

Nothing signals a little R&R more than a tropical drink. One sip transports you to a dreamy paradise where the water is turquoise and shoes are optional. When you need that moment, and the kids are playing in the backyard or swimming in the pool, find a sunny spot on your patio, put your feet up, and escape with my slimmed-down tropical refresher. This drink is a source of bromelain, an enzyme in pineapple that's a natural anti-inflammatory, digestive aid and cancer fighter. With less than 200 calories, lots of vitamin C and a mega dose of taste, this drink will have you feeling fine in no time!

YIELD: 1 serving | **TIME:** 5 minutes

⅓ cup/55 g finely chopped fresh pineapple

⅓ cup/50 g sliced banana

3 tbsp/45 ml rum

Ice cubes

1 pineapple chunk, for garnish

Place all ingredients except the garnish in a blender with a few cubes of ice. Purée until smooth. Pour into a highball glass. Garnish with pineapple chunk on the edge of the glass.

PER SERVING: Calories 170, protein 1 g, total fat 0 g, carbohydrates 18 g, sodium 0 mg, fiber 1 g

TINA'S TIP: Feel free to add a splash of light coconut milk for extra flavor and bone-building phosphorous. If you have leftover pineapple, use it to top pancakes and waffles, toss chunks into a smoothie, make quick bread and muffins, whip up some pineapple pork or grill it and serve it with a scoop of coconut sorbet.

References

Adolphe JL, Whiting SJ, Juurlink BH, et al. (2010) "Health Effects with Consumption of the Flax Lignan Secoisolariciresinol Diglucoside." *Br J Nutr.* 103(7):929-38. Retrieved from www.ncbi.nlm.nih.gov/pubmed/20003621.

Ahmed T, Sadia H, Batool S, et al. (2010) "Use of Prunes as a Control of Hypertension." *J Ayub Med Coll Abbottabad* 22(1):28-31. Retrieved from www.ncbi.nlm.nih.gov/pubmed/21409897.

Al-Shahib W, Marshall RJ. (2003) "The Fruit of the Date Palm: Its Possible Use as the Best Food for the Future?" *Int J Food Sci Nutr.* 54(4):247-59. Retrieved from www.ncbi.nlm.nih.gov/pubmed/12850886

Amarasiri WA, Dissanayake AS. (2006) "Coconut Fats." *Ceylon Med J.* 2:47-51. Retrieved from www.ncbi.nlm.nih.gov/pubmed/17180807.

Atsuko N, Takashi T, Hideaki H. (2011) "*Ipomoea batatas* and *Agaricus blazei* Ameliorate Diabetic Disorders with Therapeutic Antioxidant Potential in Streptozotocin-Induced Diabetic Rats." *J Clin Biochem Nutr.* 194–202. Epub 2011 January 7. Retrieved from www.ncbi.nlm.nih.gov/pmc/articles/PMC3082073.

Brandolini A, Hidalgo A. (2011) "Wheat Germ: Not Only a By-Product." *Int J Food Sci Nutr.* 2012 Mar;63 Suppl 1:71-4. Retrieved from www.ncbi.nlm.nih.gov/pubmed/22077851.

Campbell WW. (2007) "Protein Intake during Energy Restriction: Effects on Body Composition and Markers of Metabolic and Cardiovascular Health in Postmenopausal Women." *Journal of the American College of Nutrition.* Retrieved from www.jacn.org/content/26/2/182.full?sid=5cd29dc7-2fe9-439f-a71c-30050deb2bfe.

Carlsen MH, Halvorsen BL, Holte K, et al. (2010) "The Total Antioxidant Content of More than 3100 Foods, Beverages, Spices, Herbs and Supplements Used Worldwide." *Nutr J.* 9: 3. Epub 2010 January 22. Retrieved from www.ncbi.nlm.nih.gov/pmc/articles/PMC2841576.

Carson, Tara. (2011) "What Are the Health Benefits of Couscous?" Article reviewed by Eric Lochridge. Last updated on May 12, 2011. Retrieved from www.livestrong.com/article/440051-what-are-the-health-benefits-of-couscous.

Caselato-Sousa VM, Amaya-Farfán J. (2012) "State of Knowledge on Amaranth Grain: A Comprehensive Review." *J Food Sci.* 77(4):R93-104. Retrieved from www.ncbi.nlm.nih.gov/pubmed/22515252.

Chai SC, Hooshmand S, Saadat RL, et al. (2012) "Daily Apple versus Dried Plum: Impact on Cardiovascular Disease Risk Factors in Postmenopausal Women." *Journal of the Academy of Nutrition and Dietetics.* Epub July 26, 2012. Retrieved from www.ncbi.nlm.nih.gov/pubmed-health/behindtheheadlines/news/2012-07-27-two-apples-a-day-keeps-heart-doctor-away.

Christen WG, Liu S, Glynn RJ, et al. (2008) "Dietary Carotenoids, Vitamins C and E, and Risk of Cataract in Women: A Prospective Study." *Arch Ophthalmol.* 126(1):102-9. Retrieved from www.ncbi.nlm.nih.gov/pubmed/18195226.

Cohen EEW, Wu K, Hartford C, et al. (2012) "Phase I Studies of Sirolimus Alone or in Combination with Pharmacokinetic Modulators in Advanced Cancer Patients." *Clinical Cancer Research.* Epub August 7, 2012. Retrieved from www.ncbi.nlm.nih.gov/pubmedhealth/behindtheheadlines/news/2012-08-08-grapefruit-juice-boost-cancer-drugs.

Cossu A, Posadino AM, Giordo R, Emanueli C, Sanguinetti AM, Piscopo A, et al. (2012) "Apricot Melanoidins Prevent Oxidative Endothelial Cell Death by Counteracting Mitochondrial Oxidation and Membrane Depolarization." *PLoS One* 7(11): e48817. Retrieved from www.ncbi.nlm.nih.gov/pmc/articles/PMC3493606.

Coulman KD, Liu Z, Michaelides J, et al. (2009) "Fatty Acids and Lignans in Unground Whole Flaxseed and Sesame Seed Are Bioavailable But Have Minimal Antioxidant and Lipid-Lowering Effects in Postmenopausal Women." *Mol Nutr Food Res.* 53(11):1366-75. Retrieved from www.ncbi.nlm.nih.gov/pubmed/19824016.

Covas MI, Konstantinidou V, Fitó M. (2009) "Olive Oil and Cardiovascular Health." *J Cardiovasc Pharmacol.* 54(6):477-82. Retrieved from www.ncbi.nlm.nih.gov/pubmed/19858733.

Dahl WJ, Foster LM, Tyler RT. (2012) "Review of the Health Benefits of Peas (*Pisum sativum L.*)." Br *J Nutr.* 108 Suppl 1:S3-10. Retrieved from www.ncbi.nlm.nih.gov/pubmed/22916813.

Daley CA, Abbott A, Doyle PS, et al. (2010) "A Review of Fatty Acid Profiles and Antioxidant Content in Grass-fed and Grain-fed Beef." *Nutr. J.* Epub 2010 March 10. Retrieved from www.ncbi.nlm.nih.gov/pmc/articles/PMC2846864.

De Pascual-Teresa S, Moreno DA, Garcia-Viguera C. (2010) "Flavanols and Anthocyanins in Cardiovascular Health: A Review of Current Evidence." *Int J Mol Sci.* Epub 2010 April 13. Retrieved from www.ncbi.nlm.nih.gov/pmc/articles/PMC2871133.

Dorman K. (2011) "What Are the Benefits of Eating Beet Greens?" Article reviewed by V. Mac. Last updated on August 6, 2011. Retrieved from www.livestrong.com/article/509649-what-are-the-benefits-of-eating-beet-greens/#ixzz2CuELagFL.

Douglas SM, Ortinau LC, Hoertel HA, Leidy HJ. (2012) "Low, Moderate, or High Protein Yogurt Snacks on Appetite Control and Subsequent Eating in Healthy Women." *Appetite.* Retrieved from www.ncbi.nlm.nih.gov/pubmed/23022602.

Edwards AJ, Vinyard BT, Wiley ER, et al. (2003) "Consumption of Watermelon Juice Increases Plasma Concentrations of Lycopene and Beta-Carotene in Humans." *J Nutr.* 133(4):1043-50. Retrieved from www.ncbi.nlm.nih.gov/pubmed/12672916.

Engelmann NJ, Clinton SK, Erdman JW Jr. (2011) "Nutritional Aspects of Phytoene and Phytofluene, Carotenoid Precursors to Lycopene." *Advanced Nutrition.* 2(1): 51–61. Retrieved from www.ncbi.nlm.nih.gov/pmc/articles/PMC3042793.

Feghali K, Feldman M, La VD, et al. (2011) "Cranberry Proanthocyanidins: Natural Weapons against Periodontal Diseases." *J Agric Food Chem.* Retrieved from www.ncbi.nlm.nih.gov/pubmed/22082264.

Foran JA, Good DH, Carpenter DO, et al. (2005) "Quantitative Analysis of the Benefits and Risks of Consuming Farmed and Wild Salmon." *J Nutr.* 135(11):2639-43. Retrieved from www.ncbi.nlm.nih.gov/pubmed/16251623.

"Garlic." (2012) *Medline Plus.* U.S. National Library of Medicine, Bethesda, MD. U.S. Department of Health and Human Services, National Institutes of Health. Last Reviewed December 24, 2012. Retrieved from www.nlm.nih.gov/medlineplus/druginfo/natural/300.html.

Hong YJ, Barrett DM, Mitchell AE. (2007) "Liquid Chromatography/Mass Spectrometry Investigation of the Impact of Thermal Processing and Storage on Peach Procyanidins." *J Agric Food Chem.* 52(8):2366-71. Retrieved from www.ncbi.nlm.nih.gov/pubmed/15080647.

Illian TG, Casey JC, Bishop PA. (2011) "Omega-3 Chia Seed Loading as a Means of Carbohydrate Loading." *J Strength Cond Res.* 25(1):61-5. Retrieved from www.ncbi.nlm.nih.gov/pubmed/21183832.

Kamil A, Chen CY. (2012) "Health Benefits of Almonds beyond Cholesterol Reduction." *J Agric Food Chem.* Retrieved from www.ncbi.nlm.nih.gov/pubmed/22296169.

Kaume L, Howard LR, Devareddy L. (2011) "The Blackberry Fruit: A Review on Its Composition and Chemistry, Metabolism and Bioavailability, and Health Benefits." *J Agric Food Chem.* Retrieved from www.ncbi.nlm.nih.gov/pubmed/22082199.

Kendall CWC, Emam A, Augustin LSA, et al. (2004) "Resistant Starches and Health." *Journal of AOA International* 87(3):769-774. Retrieved from www.ingentaconnect.com/content/aoac/jaoac/2004/00000087/00000003/art00028.

Kouba M, Mourot J. (2011) "A Review of Nutritional Effects on Fat Composition of Animal Products with Special Emphasis on n-3 Polyunsaturated Fatty Acids." *Biochimie.* 93(1):13-7. Retrieved from www.ncbi.nlm.nih.gov/pubmed/20188790.

Latté KP, Appel KE, Lampen A. (2011) "Health Benefits and Possible Risks of Broccoli: An Overview." *Food Chem Toxicol.* 2011 Dec;49(12):3287-309. Retrieved from www.ncbi.nlm.nih.gov/pubmed/21906651.

Lima-Silva V, Rosado A, Amorim-Silva V, et al. (2012) "Genetic and Genome-wide Transcriptomic Analyses Identify Co-regulation of Oxidative Response and Hormone Transcript Abundance with Vitamin C Content in Tomato Fruit." *BMC Genomics.* Retrieved from www.ncbi.nlm.nih.gov/pmc/articles/PMC3462723.

Liu M, Li XQ, Weber C, et al. (2007) "Antioxidant and Antiproliferative Activities of Raspberries." *J Agric Food Chem.* 50(10):2926-30. Retrieved November 18, 2012 from www.ncbi.nlm.nih.gov/pubmed/11982421.

Lu QY, Zhang Y, Wang Y, et al. (2009) "California Hass Avocado: Profiling of Carotenoids, Tocopherol, Fatty Acid, and Fat Content During Maturation and from Different Growing Areas." *J Agric Food Chem* 57(21):10408-13. Retrieved from www.ncbi.nlm.nih.gov/pubmed/19813713.

Lu S, Van Eck J, Zhou X, et al. (2008) "The Cauliflower *Or* Gene Encodes a DnaJ Cysteine-Rich Domain-Containing Protein That Mediates High Levels of ß-Carotene Accumulation." *Plant Cell.* 3594–3605. Retrieved from www.ncbi.nlm.nih.gov/pmc/articles/PMC1785402.

Ma C, Dastmalchi K, Whitaker BD, Kennelly EJ. (2011) "Two New Antioxidant Malonated Caffeoylquinic Acid Isomers in Fruits of Wild Eggplant Relatives." *J Agric Food Chem.* 14;59(17):9645-51. Retrieved from www.ncbi.nlm.nih.gov/pubmed?term=Ma%20C%5BAuthor%5D&cauthor=true&cauthor_uid=21800866.

McCune LM, Kubota C, Stendell-Hollis NR, Thomson CA. (2011) "Cherries and Health: A Review." *Crit Rev Food Sci Nutr.* 51(1):1-12. Retrieved from www.ncbi.nlm.nih.gov/pubmed/21229414.

McKay DL, Blumberg JB. (2006) "A Review of the Bioactivity and Potential Health Benefits of Peppermint Tea (*Mentha piperita L.*)." *Phytother Res.* 20(8):619-33. Retrieved from www.ncbi.nlm.nih.gov/pubmed/16767798.

Messina M, Wu AH. (2009) "Prospectives on the Soy Breast Cancer Relationship." *Am J. Clin Nutr.* Retrieved from www.ncbi.nlm.nih.gov/pubmed/19339397.

Miller JB, Pang E, Bramall L. (1992) "Rice: A High or Low Glycemic Index Food?" *Am J. Clin Nutr.* Retrieved from http://ajcn.nutrition.org/content/56/6/1034.abstract.

Norton, Kyle J. "The World's Most Healthy Foods: Vegetable—Squash (Cucurbita) Health Benefits and Side Effects." (2011) Retrieved from http://medicaladvisorjournals.blogspot.ca/2011/12/world-most-healthy-foods-vegetable.html.

Odabasi E, Turan M, Aydin A, et al. (2008) "Magnesium, Zinc, Copper, Manganese, and Selenium Levels in Postmenopausal Women with Osteoporosis. Can Magnesium Play a Key Role in Osteoporosis?" *Ann Acad Med Singapore.* 564-7. Retrieved from www.ncbi.nlm.nih.gov/pubmed/18695768.

"Paint Your Plate with Color." (2008) Academy of Nutrition and Dietetics. Retrieved from www.eatright.org/Public/content.aspx?id=97&terms=health+benefits+of+beets#.UK147-uhD9A.

Pilon G, Ruzzin J, Rioux LE, et al. (2011) "Differential Effects of Various Fish Proteins in Altering Body Weight, Adiposity, Inflammatory Status, and Insulin Sensitivity in High-Fat-Fed Rats." *Metabolism.* 60(8):1122-30. Retrieved from www.ncbi.nlm.nih.gov/pubmed/21306751.

Ros, Emilio. (2010) "Health Benefits of Nut Consumption." *Nutrients.* 2(7):652–682. Retrieved from www.ncbi.nlm.nih.gov/pmc/articles/PMC3257681.

Sabater-Molina M, Larqué E, Torrella F, Zamora S. (2009) "Dietary Fructooligosaccharides and Potential Benefits on Health." *J Physiol Biochem.*65 (3):315-28. Retrieved from www.ncbi.nlm.nih.gov/pubmed/20119826.

Sowbhagya HB. (2013) "Chemistry, Technology, and Nutraceutical Functions of Cumin (*Cuminum cyminum L*): An Overview." *Crit Rev Food Sci Nutr* 53(1):1-10 Retrieved from www.ncbi.nlm.nih.gov/pubmed/23035918.

Tiran, D. (2012) "Ginger to Reduce Nausea and Vomiting During Pregnancy: Evidence of Effectiveness Is Not the Same as Proof of Safety." *Complement Ther Clin Pract.* 18(1):22-5. Retrieved from www.ncbi.nlm.nih.gov/pubmed/22196569.

Vinson JA, Cai Y. (2012) "Nuts, Especially Walnuts, Have Both Antioxidant Quantity and Efficacy and Exhibit Significant Potential Health Benefits." *Food Funct.* Retrieved from www.ncbi.nlm.nih.gov/pubmed/22187094.

Vinson JA, Zubik L, Bose P, et al. (2005) "Dried Fruits: Excellent in Vitro and in Vivo Antioxidants." *J Am Coll Nutr.* Retrieved from www.jacn.org/content/24/1/44.full.

Wenche F, Åman P. (2010) "Whole Grain for Whom and Why?" *Food Nutr Res.* Retrieved from www.ncbi.nlm.nih.gov/pmc/articles/PMC2840227.

Wilson RD, Davies G, Désilets V, et al. (2003) "The Use of Folic Acid for the Prevention of Neural Tube Defects and Other Congenital Anomalies." *J Obstet Gynaecol Can.* (11):959-73. Retrieved from www.ncbi.nlm.nih.gov/pubmed/14608448.

Winham DM, Hutchins AM. (2011) "Perceptions of Flatulence from Bean Consumption among Adults in 3 Feeding Studies." *Nutr J.* 10:128. Retrieved from www.ncbi.nlm.nih.gov/pubmed/22104320.

Yun YS, Noda S, Shigemori G, et al. (2012) "Phenolic Diterpenes from Rosemary Suppress cAMP Responsiveness of Gluconeogenic Gene Promoters." *Phytother Res.* Retrieved from www.ncbi.nlm.nih.gov/pubmed/22927089.

Zhang Y, Suk Jung C, De Jong WS. (2009) "Genetic Analysis of Pigmented Tuber Flesh in Potato." *Theor Appl Genet.* 119(1): 143–150. Retrieved from www.ncbi.nlm.nih.gov/pmc/articles/PMC2690854.

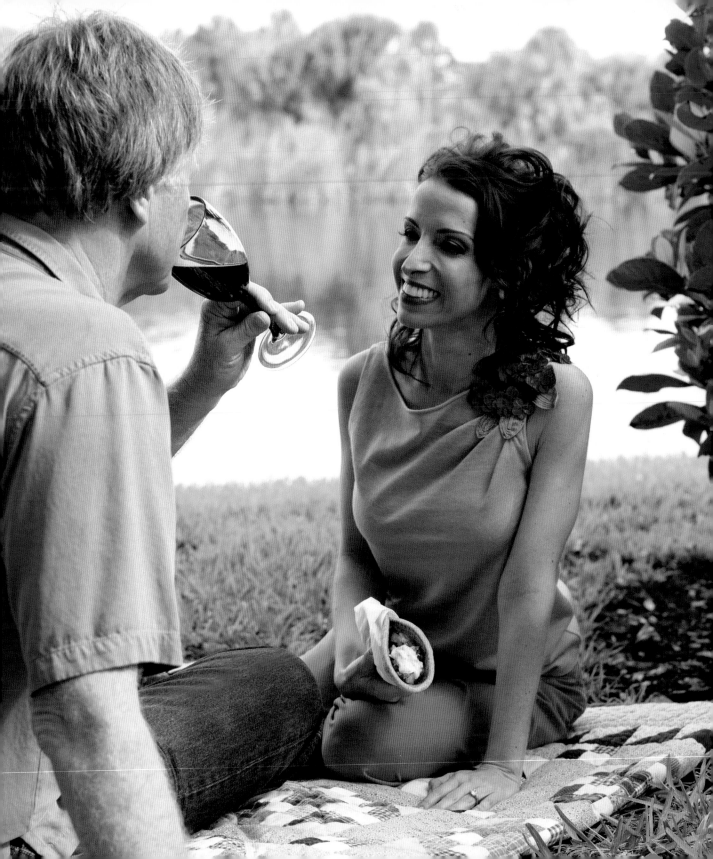

Acknowledgements

Years of experience as a nutritionist, cook, writer and food stylist have culminated in this book. My hope is that within these pages you can see and feel the enthusiasm I have for healthy, delicious cooking. Of course, communicating my intent would not be possible without a team of talented, smart and dedicated professionals who took the creation and development of this book as seriously as I did.

Thank you to my publisher, Will Kiester, for sharing my vision, allowing me to freely ideate and giving me the creative liberty to help produce a book that filled a void. To my mother, who worked with me side by side, testing and retesting (and sometimes testing again) my recipe concepts. I'm in debt to her for her insight, opinion, experience and, of course, for washing about 5,000 dishes. Thanks, Mom, for the laughs and the memories! To my dad, my super-taster, offering spot-on critiques and contributing to creative development. You are an ace with names! To Richard, my quiet, compassionate husband whose patience, support and love are constant. And to my aunt Yvonne, for her never-ending interest, enthusiasm, love and inspiration.

I'd also like to thank my team of modern-day Wonder Women: Andrea Lynn, KT McNamara, Amy and Mia Galvin and Abigail Hitchcock, for tasting, testing, advising and believing in my project.

My sincere thanks to Bill and Gwynne Bettencourt. What a pleasure it was working with such a talented team. I'm so grateful for your collaboration.

Last, and certainly not least, to all of my friends, who were understanding when writing and cooking consumed me, and I had to decline lunch dates, lessons, dinners, workouts, parties … Thank you for your support and for your loyal friendship. I could not have written this book without your continuous encouragement and belief in my purpose.

Recipe Index

Note: Page numbers in italics indicate photographs.

A
All-Star Kale and Potato Frittata, *28*, 29
Angel's Slice, 155
The Apple of My Eye, *146*, 147
Autumn Harvest Pasta, 93

B
"Belgian" Slaw, 129
Best Pesto Scramble, 43
Beyond Belief, 92
Blueberry Cassis Fizz, 196
Boost-My-Mood Banana Smoothie, 31
Bundles of Joy, 109
Butternut Squash Mix 'n' Mash, 160

C
Can't Beet This, 117
Caribbean Sammy, 56
Charming Charmoula, 88
Chicken Salad Sammy, 48, *49*
Chocolate Peanut Butter Power Bites, 176
Chow These Chops, 68, *69*
Confetti Farfalle, *120*, 121
Cozy Comfort Bread Pudding, 144
Creamy Dreamy Orange Tea, 188

D
Desert Song, 77
Do the Salmon Slide, *80*, 81
Double Dippin' Delights, 154
Dynamite Egg Poppers, 169

E
Earl Grey Pear Latte, 189
Easy Breezy Island Tacos, 86, *87*

F
Farmer's Harvest, 128

Fish in Paradise, 85
Flip for Flapjacks, 20
Flipped-Out Flapjacks, 166, *167*
Full 'n' Plenty, 64

G
Get Figgie With It, 103
Get Your Jam On, 53
Ginger Rogers, 197
Green Eggs and Ham Torpedo, 33

H
Happy Veggie Pocket, 59
Heart Throb, 136, *137*
Hibiscus-Ginger Refresher, 190, *191*
Homemade Holiday Hit, 71
Honolulu Breeze, 199
Hot Mama, 78, *79*

I
Irresistible Almond-Garlic Dip, 175
Italian Rice Is Nice, 101

K
Keep Your Eye on the Pizza Pie, 107
Kippers and Bits, 60, *61*
Kiss My Cakes, 26, *27*

L
The Lean Machine, *72*, 73
Let's Roll, 165
Little Miss Savory Muffins, 23
Lovin' Spoonful, 34

M
Make My Date (Date and Almond Muffins), 32
Make My Meatballs, 74
The Marvelous Mediterranean, 113
Meatless Madness, 112
The Meatless Mediterranean, 83

Mighty Melon-Berry Float, 156, *157*
"Min-Tea" Energizer, *192*, 193
Mixed Bag, 125
Mix It Up Müesli, 18, *19*
Mother Nature's Green Machine, 35

N
Naturally Nutritious Power Bars, 180
New Dehli Belly, 47
Not Mean Greens, 124

O
Oh, My! Spaghetti Surprise, 67
Oodles of Noodles Salad, 139
Orange Vodka Snowball, 194
Orange You Fabulous, 38
Oui, Oui, Mon Cherie!, 122
Over the Rainbow, *152*, 153

P
Parma Panini, 55
Peachy Pork, 65
Perfect Pumpkin Soup, 97
Pickle My Fancy, *172*, 173
Pop-in-Your-Mouth PB&J Bites, 149
Power Nutrient Parfait, 30
Power Pesto, 96
Presto Pesto Bean Dip, 170, *171*

Q
Quinoa Tabbouleh, 126

R
Raspberry Coulis, 143
Rat-a-Tat-Tat, 108
Razzle Dazzle Berry Mocha, 185
Rev Up 'n' Go Baked Eggs, 24
Rising Sun Pork Bun, 51
Roll Model, 179
Rosie's Better Beans, 119

S
Savory Sea Veggie Salad, 118
The Scandalous Scandinavian, 51
See Food Your Way, 104
Shrimp on a Limb, 164
Siesta Special, 135

Silly Fusilli, *110*, 111
Simply Peachy, 39
Simply Savory Stuffed Pork, 70
Skinny Cheesecake Minis, 142
South-of-the-Border Soother, 184
Spanish Eyes, 106
Spice Is Nice!, *186*, 187
Spin the Wheel, 89
Squeeze Me!, 50
A Star Is Born Popcorn, 161
Star-Studded Black Rice, 131
Strawberries on a Cloud, *162*, 163
Sunday Special, 40, *41*
Superberry Smoothie, 25
Super Simple Sensation, 84

T
The Tahini Thrill, 123
Take-Me-Away Tropical Fruit Smoothie, 42
Tasty Trio, 58
The Three Musketeers, 82
Three Times the Charm, 95
Tina's Famous Farro, 134
Tuna Tune-Up, 57
Tuscan Winter Warmer, 102
Tutti Fruitti, 21
Two to Tango, 46

V
Veggie Nice Salad, 132, *133*
Velvety Veggie Mac 'n' Cheese, 98, *99*

W
Wild about Veggies, 116
Wok This Way, 75

Y
Yam, Yam Good!, 138
Yummy Chunky Chocolate Brownies, 150, *151*

Z
Zorba the Greek, 76

Index

A

adobo sauce, 78

agave nectar, 35

alfalfa sprouts, 59

almond butter, 31

almond milk, 18

almonds

Can't Beet This, 117

Cozy Comfort Bread Pudding, 144

Farmer's Harvest, 128

Irresistible Almond-Garlic Dip, 175

Make My Date, 32

Not Mean Greens, 124

amaretto liqueur, 34

anchovies, 136

apples, 18, 20

The Apple of My Eye, 147

"Belgian" Slaw, 129

Love Me, Love My Smoothie, 37

Two to Tango, 46

apricots

Desert Song, 77

Double Dippin' Delights, 154

Make My Meatballs, 74

Naturally Nutritious Power Bars, 180

Power Nutrient Parfait, 30

artichokes, 113

arugula

Chicken Salad Sammy, 48

Get Figgie With It, 103

Keep Your Eye on the Pizza Pie, 107

Mixed Bag, 125

Strawberries on a Cloud, 163

asparagus

Squeeze Me!, 50

Super Simple Sensation, 84

Wild about Veggies, 116

avocados

Caribbean Sammy, 56

Fish in Paradise, 85

Kippers and Bits, 60

Quinoa Tabbouleh, 126

Savory Sea Veggie Salad, 118

Siesta Special, 135

B

bacon. *See* turkey bacon

balsamic vinegar, 103, 107, 128, 163

bananas

Honolulu Breeze, 199

Superberry Smoothie, 31

Take-Me-Away Tropical Fruit Smoothie, 42

Tasty Trio, 58

bars, 180

basil

"Belgian" Slaw, 129

Best Pesto Scramble, 43

Confetti Farfalle, 121

The Meatless Mediterranean, 83

Power Pesto, 96

Rat-a-Tat-Tat, 108

Shrimp on a Limb, 164

Squeeze Me!, 50

Strawberries on a Cloud, 163

Veggie Nice Salad, 132

bay leaves
Beyond Belief, 92
Pickle My Fancy, 173
bean dip, 170
beans
black beans, 56, 92, 135
butter beans, 119
cannelini beans, 102
gigante beans, 102
green beans, 111, 125
lima beans, 102
pinto beans, 106
white beans, 170
bean sprouts, 86
beef
Homemade Holiday Hit, 71
The Lean Machine, 73
Make My Meatballs, 74
Saucy Beef Bonbons, 174
Wok This Way, 75
beet greens
Can't Beet This, 117
Dynamite Egg Poppers, 169
beets
Autumn Harvest Pasta, 93
Can't Beet This, 117
Chow These Chops, 68
Pickle My Fancy, 173
Veggie Nice Salad, 132
beverages, 183–99
Blueberry Cassis Fizz, 196
Boost-My-Mood Banana Smoothie, 31
Creamy Dreamy Orange Tea, 188
floats, 156
Ginger Rogers, 197
Hibiscus-Ginger Refresher, 190
Honolulu Breeze, 199
hot cocoa, 184

Love Me, Love My Smoothie, 37
Mighty Melon-Berry Float, 156
"Min-Tea" Energizer, 193
mocha, 185
Orange Vodka Snowball, 194
Razzle Dazzle Berry Mocha, 185
smoothies, 25, 31, 42
South-of-the-Border Soother, 184
Spice Is Nice!, 187
Superberry Smoothie, 25
Take-Me-Away Tropical Fruit Smoothie, 42
black beans
Beyond Belief, 92
Caribbean Sammy, 56
Meatless Madness, 112
Siesta Special, 135
blackberries, 82
blueberries
Blueberry Cassis Fizz, 196
Kiss My Cakes, 26
Superberry Smoothie, 31
Tutti Fruitti, 21
Whey to Go Yogurt Brûlée, 148
bok choy, 75
bouillabaisse, 104
bread, 40, 47, 98, 144. *See also* sandwiches
bread puddings, 144
breakfast, 17–44
All-Star Kale and Potato Frittata, 29
Best Pesto Scramble, 43
Boost-My-Mood Banana Smoothie, 31
Flip for Flapjacks, 20
Green Eggs and Ham Torpedo, 33
Kiss My Cakes, 26
Little Miss Savory Muffins, 23
Love Me, Love My Smoothie, 37
Lovin' Spoonful, 34
Make My Date, 32

breakfast, continued

    Mix It Up Müesli, 18

    Mother Nature's Green Machine, 35

    Orange You Fabulous, 38

    Power Nutrient Parfait, 30

    Rev Up 'n' Go Baked Eggs, 24

    Simply Peachy, 39

    smoothies, 35, 37

    Sunday Special, 40

    Superberry Smoothie, 25

    Tutti Fruitti, 21

brie, 103

brioche, 144

broccoli

    Presto Pesto Bean Dip, 170

    Velvety Veggie Mac 'n' Cheese, 98

broccoli rabe, 113

brownies, 150

brown sugar, 34

brunch, 17–44

Brussels sprouts

    "Belgian" Slaw, 129

    Autumn Harvest Pasta, 93

bulgur, 108

burgers

    Do the Salmon Slide, 81

    The Lean Machine, 73

    Meatless Madness, 112

    Zorba the Greek, 76

burritos, Green Eggs and Ham Torpedo, 33

butter beans, 119

buttermilk, 155

butternut squash

    Butternut Squash Mix 'n' Mash, 160

    Italian Rice Is Nice, 101

    Perfect Pumpkin Soup, 97

    Tina's Famous Farro, 134

C

cakes

    Angel's Slice, 155

    Skinny Cheesecake Minis, 142

cannelini beans, 102

capers, 52, 83

carrots

    Desert Song, 77

    Easy Breezy Island Tacos, 86

    Flipped-Out Flapjacks, 166

    Happy Veggie Pocket, 59

    Oodles of Noodles Salad, 139

    Pickle My Fancy, 173

    Savory Sea Veggie Salad, 118

    Super Simple Sensation, 84

cassis (crème de), 196

cauliflower, 173

celery

    Love Me, Love My Smoothie, 37

    Pickle My Fancy, 173

cereal, 18

challah, 144

chard

    Bundles of Joy, 109

    Simply Savory Stuffed Pork, 70

    Tina's Famous Farro, 134

Cheddar cheese

    Get Your Jam On, 53

    Little Miss Savory Muffins, 23

    Two to Tango, 46

cheese

    brie, 103

    Cheddar cheese, 23, 46, 53, 98

    feta cheese, 109, 177

    fontina cheese, 24

    goat cheese, 169

    Gorgonzola cheese, 107, 125

    Gruyère cheese, 55

    mozzarella cheese, 33, 50, 95

Parmigiano-Reggiano cheese, 29, 64, 67, 70, 95, 98, 101, 102, 108, 111, 113, 129, 160, 161, 163, 174

Provolone cheese, 73

ricotta cheese, 40, 64, 93, 95, 107, 113, 163

ricotta salata cheese, 132

Velvety Veggie Mac 'n' Cheese, 98

cheesecakes, 142

cherries

Chocolate Peanut Butter Power Bites, 176

Desert Song, 77

Heart Throb, 136

Orange You Fabulous, 38

Sunday Special, 40

chia seeds, 149

Siesta Special, 135

chicken

Chicken Salad Sammy, 48

Desert Song, 77

Full 'n' Plenty, 64

See Food Your Way, 106

Star-Studded Black Rice, 131

chicken salad, 48

chicken sausage, 67

chicken tagine, 77

chickpeas

Beyond Belief, 92

Happy Veggie Pocket, 59

chiles, 92, 106. See also chipotles in adobo; jalapeño peppers

chili powder, 92

chipotles in adobo

Beyond Belief, 92

Hot Mama, 78

Meatless Madness, 112

Two to Tango, 46

chives, 97

chocolate. See also cocoa powder

Angel's Slice, 155

Chocolate Peanut Butter Power Bites, 176

Double Dippin' Delights, 154

Tasty Trio, 58

Whey to Go Yogurt Brûlée, 148

Yummy Chunky Chocolate Brownies, 150

chocolate-hazelnut spread, 58

chutney, 65

cider vinegar, 65

cilantro

Beyond Belief, 92

Caribbean Sammy, 56

Charming Charmoula, 88

Do the Salmon Slide, 81

Meatless Madness, 112

New Dehli Belly, 47

See Food Your Way, 106

Siesta Special, 135

cinnamon

Desert Song, 77

Earl Grey Pear Latte, 189

Easy Breezy Island Tacos, 86

Make My Date, 32

South-of-the-Border Soother, 184

Spice is Nice!, 187

Sunday Special, 40

Tutti Fruitti, 21

clams, 104

cocoa powder

Angel's Slice, 155

Chocolate Peanut Butter Power Bites, 176

Razzle Dazzle Berry Mocha, 185

South-of-the-Border Soother, 184

Yummy Chunky Chocolate Brownies, 150

coconut

Chocolate Peanut Butter Power Bites, 176

Naturally Nutritious Power Bars, 180

coconut milk, 42

cod

Fish in Paradise, 85

The Meatless Mediterranean, 83

coffee
    Orange Vodka Snowball, 194
    Razzle Dazzle Berry Mocha, 185
    South-of-the-Border Soother, 184
    Spice Is Nice!, 187
condiments
    Irresistible Almond-Garlic Dip, 175
    Power Pesto, 96
    Presto Pesto Bean Dip, 170
    Scoop My Salsa, 177
coriander
    Desert Song, 77
    Do the Salmon Slide, 81
    Zorba the Greek, 76
coriander seeds, 173
corn
    Confetti Farfalle, 121
    Farmer's Harvest, 128
corncakes, 26
cornmeal, 107
couscous
    Bundles of Joy, 109
    Desert Song, 77
    Make My Meatballs, 74
    Mixed Bag, 125
    Orange You Fabulous, 38
cranberries
    Desert Song, 77
    Homemade Holiday Hit, 71
    Tina's Famous Farro, 134
cranberry juice, 196
cream cheese, 142
cremini mushrooms, 71, 89
    Italian Rice Is Nice, 101
cucumbers
    Do the Salmon Slide, 81
    Happy Veggie Pocket, 59
    Love Me, Love My Smoothie, 37
    Make My Meatballs, 74

New Dehli Belly, 47
Oodles of Noodles Salad, 139
Pickle My Fancy, 173
Quinoa Tabbouleh, 126
Savory Sea Veggie Salad, 118
Scoop My Salsa, 177
Zorba the Greek, 76
cumin
    Bundles of Joy, 109
    Caribbean Sammy, 56
    Desert Song, 77
    Meatless Madness, 112
    Peachy Pork, 65
    The Tahini Thrill, 123
    Two to Tango, 46
    Zorba the Greek, 76
curry paste, 81
curry powder, 166
    New Dehli Belly, 47

D
dates
    Desert Song, 77
    Make My Date, 32
desserts, 141–58
    Angel's Slice, 155
    The Apple of My Eye, 147
    Chocolate Peanut Butter Power Bites, 176
    Cozy Comfort Bread Pudding, 144
    Double Dippin' Delights, 154
    Mighty Melon-Berry Float, 156
    Over the Rainbow, 153
    Pop-in-Your-Mouth PB&J Bites, 149
    popsicles, 153
    Raspberry Coulis, 143
    Skinny Cheesecake Minis, 142
    Whey to Go Yogurt Brûlée, 148
    Yummy Chunky Chocolate Brownies, 150
Dijon mustard, 122, 128, 163

dill
>Chicken Salad Sammy, 48
>Pickle My Fancy, 173
>The Scandalous Scandinavian, 52

dips
>Irresistible Almond-Garlic Dip, 175
>Presto Pesto Bean Dip, 170
>Scoop My Salsa, 177

dried fruit, 77, 180

E

edadame, 121

eggplant
>Rat-a-Tat-Tat, 108
>The Tahini Thrill, 123

eggs
>All-Star Kale and Potato Frittata, 29
>Best Pesto Scramble, 43
>Dynamite Egg Poppers, 169
>Flipped-Out Flapjacks, 166
>Green Eggs and Ham Torpedo, 33
>Hot Mama, 78
>Rev Up 'n' Go Baked Eggs, 24
>The Scandalous Scandinavian, 52
>Simply Savory Stuffed Pork, 70
>Sunday Special, 40
>Tuna Tune-Up, 57
>Yummy Chunky Chocolate Brownies, 150

F

farfalle, 93

fennel, 57

fennel seeds, 93

feta cheese
>Bundles of Joy, 109
>Scoop My Salsa, 177

fettuccine, The Marvelous Mediterranean, 113

figs, 103

fish
>anchovies, 136
>Charming Charmoula, 88
>cod, 83, 85
>en papillote, 84
>Fish in Paradise, 85
>grouper, 83
>haddock, 83, 88, 89
>kippers, 60
>The Meatless Mediterranean, 83
>perch, 83
>red snapper, 83
>salmon, 52, 81, 82, 84
>snapper, 83
>Spin the Wheel, 89
>Super Simple Sensation, 84
>The Three Musketeers, 82
>tuna, 57

fish sauce, 81

fish stock, 104

flatbread, 91–114
>Get Figgie With It, 103
>Three Times the Charm, 95

fontina cheese, 24

French toast, 40

frittatas, All-Star Kale and Potato Frittata, 29

frozen yogurt. *See* yogurt, frozen

fruit, 18, 21, 25, 58, 77, 148, 165. *See also specific fruit*

fruit salad, 21

fusilli, 111

G

garbanzo beans. *See* chickpeas

garlic
>Butternut Squash Mix 'n' Mash, 160
>Irresistible Almond-Garlic Dip, 175
>The Meatless Mediterranean, 83
>Not Mean Greens, 124
>Super Simple Sensation, 84

gigante beans, Tuscan Winter Warmer, 102

ginger

Flipped-Out Flapjacks, 166

Ginger Rogers, 197

Hibiscus-Ginger Refresher, 190

Love Me, Love My Smoothie, 37

New Dehli Belly, 47

Oodles of Noodles Salad, 139

pickled, 179

Rising Sun Pork Bun, 51

Savory Sea Veggie Salad, 118

Spice Is Nice!, 187

Super Simple Sensation, 84

goat cheese, 169

Gorgonzola cheese, 107, 125

graham crackers, 142

granola

Power Nutrient Parfait, 30

Tasty Trio, 58

granola bars, 180

grapefruit, 34

Veggie Nice Salad, 132

grapes, 18, 21, 48

grape tomatoes

Farmer's Harvest, 128

Shrimp on a Limb, 164

Greek salad, 177

Greek yogurt. *See* yogurt, Greek

green beans

Mixed Bag, 125

Silly Fusilli, 111

green bell peppers, Beyond Belief, 92

greens

Caribbean Sammy, 56

Dynamite Egg Poppers, 169

Farmer's Harvest, 128

Flipped-Out Flapjacks, 166

kippers, 60

Not Mean Greens, 124

The Scandalous Scandinavian, 52

Tuna Tune-Up, 57

Veggie Nice Salad, 132

green tea, "Min-Tea" Energizer, 193

gremolata, 111

grilled cheese sandwiches, 53

grouper, 83

Gruyère cheese, 55

H

haddock

Charming Charmoula, 88

The Meatless Mediterranean, 83

ham

Green Eggs and Ham Torpedo, 33

Parma Panini, 55

hamburgers, The Lean Machine, 73

hazelnuts, 147

hemp seeds, 95, 154

honey

Chocolate Peanut Butter Power Bites, 176

Creamy Dreamy Orange Tea, 188

Earl Grey Pear Latte, 189

Flip for Flapjacks, 20

"Min-Tea" Energizer, 193

Superberry Smoothie, 25

hot cocoa, 184

hummus, 59

J

jalapeño peppers, 35

jam, 53

jasmine rice, 75

K

kalamata olives, 177

kale

All-Star Kale and Potato Frittata, 29

Full 'n' Plenty, 64

Heart Throb, 136

Italian Rice Is Nice, 101

Love Me, Love My Smoothie, 37

Not Mean Greens, 124

Oh, My! Spaghetti Surprise, 67

Power Pesto, 96

Tuscan Winter Warmer, 102

kefir, 18

kippers, 60

kiwis, 21, 153

L

lamb burgers, 76

lattes, Earl Grey Pear Latte, 189

leeks, 89

lemon juice, 59

lemons

Blueberry Cassis Fizz, 196

Can't Beet This, 117

Quinoa Tabbouleh, 126

Simply Peachy, 39

The Tahini Thrill, 123

lettuce, *see also* arugula, mesclun

Farmer's Harvest, 128

kippers, 60

The Lean Machine, 73

Mixed Bag, 125

Roll Model, 179

Star-Studded Black Rice, 131

Zorba the Greek, 76

lima beans, 102

lime juice, 35, 42, 197

limes, 190

Little Miss Savory Muffins, *22*

Love Me, Love My Smoothie, 37

M

macaroni and cheese, 98

mangoes, 85

mango nectar, 190

maple syrup, 95

martinis, Ginger Rogers, 197

mayonnaise, 52, 60

meatballs

Make My Meatballs, 74

Saucy Beef Bonbons, 174

meatless main courses

Beyond Belief, 92

Meatless Madness, 112

The Meatless Mediterranean, 83

vegetarian chili, 92

meatloaf, Hot Mama, 78

mesclun

Farmer's Harvest, 128

Savory Sea Veggie Salad, 118

Veggie Nice Salad, 132

milk

Creamy Dreamy Orange Tea, 188

Earl Grey Pear Latte, 189

Mother Nature's Green Machine, 35

Razzle Dazzle Berry Mocha, 185

South-of-the-Border Soother, 184

Spice Is Nice!, 187

mint

Mighty Melon-Berry Float, 156

"Min-Tea" Energizer, 193

Mother Nature's Green Machine, 35

Quinoa Tabbouleh, 126

Scoop My Salsa, 177

The Tahini Thrill, 123

Take-Me-Away Tropical Fruit Smoothie, 42

Whey to Go Yogurt Brûlée, 148

mocha, Razzle Dazzle Berry Mocha, 185

molasses, 149

Mother Nature's Green Machine, *36*

mozzarella cheese

Green Eggs and Ham Torpedo, 33

Squeeze Me!, 50

Three Times the Charm, 95

müesli, 18

muffins

  Little Miss Savory Muffins, 23

  Make My Date, 32

mushrooms

  Homemade Holiday Hit, 71

  Italian Rice Is Nice, 101

  Spin the Wheel, 89

  Wild about Veggies, 116

  Wok This Way, 75

mussels, See Food Your Way, 104

mustard, 52, 122, 128, 163

mustard seeds, 173

N

naan, 47

new potatoes, 122

noodles, 139

nori, 179

Nutella, 58

nutmeg

  Spice Is Nice!, 187

  Strawberries on a Cloud, 163

  Sunday Special, 40

  Velvety Veggie Mac 'n' Cheese, 98

nuts

  almonds, 32, 117, 124, 128, 144, 175

  hazelnuts, 147

  peanuts, 180

  pecans, 18, 40

  pine nuts, 70

  walnuts, 48, 134, 136, 150, 160

O

oats

  Chocolate Peanut Butter Power Bites, 176

  Mix It Up Müesili, 18

  Naturally Nutritious Power Bars, 180

okra, 173

olive oil, 123, 160

  Quinoa Tabbouleh, 126

olives, 122, 177

one-dish wonders, 91–114

onions

  Easy Breezy Island Tacos, 86

  Fish in Paradise, 85

  Keep Your Eye on the Pizza Pie, 107

  Kippers and Bits, 60

  Make My Meatballs, 74

  The Meatless Mediterranean, 83

  Mixed Bag, 125

  Scoop My Salsa, 177

orange liqueur, Orange Vodka Snowball, 194

oranges

  Caribbean Sammy, 56

  Chow These Chops, 68

  Flip for Flapjacks, 20

  Orange Vodka Snowball, 194

  Orange You Fabulous, 38

  Sunday Special, 40

Orange Vodka Snowball, *195*

orange zest, 153, 188

orecchiette, 111

oregano

  Full 'n' Plenty, 64

  Scoop My Salsa, 177

P

pancakes

  Flip for Flapjacks, 20

  Flipped-Out Flapjacks, 165

panini, Parma Panini, 55

paprika, Easy Breezy Island Tacos, 86

Parmigiano-Reggiano cheese, 108

  All-Star Kale and Potato Frittata, 29

  "Belgian" Slaw, 129

  Butternut Squash Mix 'n' Mash, 160

  Full 'n' Plenty, 64

  Italian Rice Is Nice, 101

  The Marvelous Mediterranean, 113

  Oh, My! Spaghetti Surprise, 67

Saucy Beef Bonbons, 174

Silly Fusilli, 111

Simply Savory Stuffed Pork, 70

A Star Is Born Popcorn, 161

Strawberries on a Cloud, 163

Three Times the Charm, 95

Tuscan Winter Warmer, 102

parsley

"Belgian" Slaw, 129

Quinoa Tabbouleh, 126

pasta, 91-114

Autumn Harvest Pasta, 93

Confetti Farfalle, 121

The Marvelous Mediterranean, 113

Oh, My! Spaghetti Surprise, 67

Silly Fusilli, 111

Velvety Veggie Mac 'n' Cheese, 98

peach butter, 39

peaches

Cozy Comfort Bread Pudding, 144

Ginger Rogers, 197

Mixed Bag, 125

Parma Panini, 55

Peachy Pork, 65

Power Nutrient Parfait, 30

Simply Peachy, 39

Superberry Smoothie, 25

peach nectar, 197

peanut butter

Chocolate Peanut Butter Power Bites, 176

Oodles of Noodles Salad, 139

Pop-in-Your-Mouth PB&J Bites, 149

peanuts, 180

pears

Earl Grey Pear Latte, 189

Tasty Trio, 58

The Three Musketeers, 82

Three Times the Charm, 95

peas, 75

pecans, 18

Sunday Special, 40

pepita seeds, 138. See also pumpkin seeds

perch, 83

pesto

Best Pesto Scramble, 43

Power Pesto, 96

Presto Pesto Bean Dip, 170

Squeeze Me!, 50

pickled ginger, 179

pickles, 173

pineapple

Honolulu Breeze, 199

Over the Rainbow, 153

Take-Me-Away Tropical Fruit Smoothie, 42

pine nuts, Simply Savory Stuffed Pork, 70

pinto beans, 106

pita bread, 59, 175, 177

pizza

Get Figgie With It, 103

Keep Your Eye on the Pizza Pie, 107

Three Times the Charm, 95

plums, 30

popcorn, 161

popsicles, 153

pork

Chow These Chops, 68

Green Eggs and Ham Torpedo, 33

ham, 33, 55

Little Miss Savory Muffins, 23

Parma Panini, 55

Peachy Pork, 65

prosciutto, 23, 102

Rising Sun Pork Bun, 51

Simply Savory Stuffed Pork, 70

Tuscan Winter Warmer, 102

potatoes

All-Star Kale and Potato Frittata, 29

New Dehli Belly, 47

Oui, Oui, Mon Cherie!, 122

Silly Fusilli, 111

power bars, 180

prosciutto, 23

    Tuscan Winter Warmer, 102

protein powder, 180

proteins, 63–90

Provolone cheese, The Lean Machine, 73

prunes

    Desert Song, 77

    Yummy Chunky Chocolate Brownies, 150

pumpkin

    Perfect Pumpkin Soup, 97

    Spice Is Nice!, 187

pumpkin seeds

    Power Pesto, 96

    Yam, Yam Good!, 138

Q

quesadillas

    Tasty Trio, 58

    Two to Tango, 46

quiche, 169

quinoa

    Quinoa Tabbouleh, 126

    Roll Model, 179

R

radishes

    Extreme Makeover Chicken Salad Sammy, 48

    Pickle My Fancy, 173

raisins, 21

    Bundles of Joy, 109

    Desert Song, 77

    Peachy Pork, 65

    Simply Savory Stuffed Pork, 70

raspberries

    Cozy Comfort Bread Pudding, 144

    Raspberry Coulis, 142

    Razzle Dazzle Berry Mocha, 185

    Superberry Smoothie, 25

    Whey to Go Yogurt Brûlée, 148

ratatouille, 108

red bell peppers

    Beyond Belief, 92

    Confetti Farfalle, 121

    Oodles of Noodles Salad, 139

    Parma Panini, 55

    Simply Savory Stuffed Pork, 70

red grapes, 48

red onions

    "Belgian" Slaw, 129

    Easy Breezy Island Tacos, 86

    Fish in Paradise, 85

    Make My Meatballs, 74

    Scoop My Salsa, 177

    Veggie Nice Salad, 132

red potatoes, 29, 111

red snapper, 83

red wine vinegar, 177

rice

    Italian Rice Is Nice, 101

    Savory Sea Veggie Salad, 118

    See Food Your Way, 106

    Siesta Special, 135

    Star-Studded Black Rice, 131

    Wok This Way, 75

ricotta cheese

    Autumn Harvest Pasta, 93

    Full 'n' Plenty, 64

    Keep Your Eye on the Pizza Pie, 107

    The Marvelous Mediterranean, 113

    Strawberries on a Cloud, 163

    Sunday Special, 40

    Three Times the Charm, 95

ricotta salata cheese, 132

risotto, Italian Rice Is Nice, 101

roasted red pepper, Simply Savory Stuffed Pork, 70

roasted red peppers, Parma Panini, 55

Roll Model, *178*

romaine lettuce, 179

rosemary

Full 'n' Plenty, 64

Keep Your Eye on the Pizza Pie, 107

Power Nutrient Parfait, 30

Rosie's Better Beans, 119

A Star Is Born Popcorn, 161

Tuscan Winter Warmer, 102

rum, 199

S

saffron, 104

sage, 93

salads, 115–40

"Belgian" Slaw, 129

Farmer's Harvest, 128

Greek salad, 177

Heart Throb, 136

Mixed Bag, 125

Oodles of Noodles Salad, 139

Savory Sea Veggie Salad, 118

Scoop My Salsa, 177

Siesta Special, 135

Star-Studded Black Rice, 131

Veggie Nice Salad, 132

salmon

Do the Salmon Slide, 81

The Scandalous Scandinavian, 52

Super Simple Sensation, 84

The Three Musketeers, 82

salsa, 177

sandwiches

Caribbean Sammy, 56

Chicken Salad Sammy, 48

Do the Salmon Slide, 81

Easy Breezy Island Tacos, 86

Get Your Jam On, 53

Happy Veggie Pocket, 59

Kippers and Bits, 60

The Lean Machine, 73

New Dehli Belly, 47

Parma Panini, 55

Quinoa Tabbouleh, 126

Rising Sun Pork Bun, 51

The Scandalous Scandinavian, 52

Squeeze Me!, 50

Tasty Trio, 58

Tuna Tune-Up, 57

Two to Tango, 46

Saucy Beef Bonbons, 174

sausage, 67. *See also* chicken sausage

scallions

Chicken Salad Sammy, 48

Desert Song, 77

Do the Salmon Slide, 81

Flipped-Out Flapjacks, 166

Oodles of Noodles Salad, 139

Rising Sun Pork Bun, 51

Savory Sea Veggie Salad, 118

Star-Studded Black Rice, 131

Wok This Way, 75

scallops, See Food Your Way, 104

Scoop My Salsa, 177

scrambles, 43

seaweed

Roll Model, 179

Savory Sea Veggie Salad, 118

seeds, sunflower seeds, 180

sesame oil, 84, 118

sesame seeds, 116, 139

shallots

Confetti Farfalle, 121

Green Eggs and Ham Torpedo, 33

Homemade Holiday Hit, 71

The Lean Machine, 73

Oui, Oui, Mon Cherie!, 122

Rev Up 'n' Go Baked Eggs, 24

See Food Your Way, 104

shellfish, 104. *See also specific kinds of shellfish*

sherry vinegar, 65

shiitake mushrooms, 75

shrimp
    Caribbean Sammy, 56
    Easy Breezy Island Tacos, 86
    The Marvelous Mediterranean, 113
    Quinoa Tabbouleh, 126
    See Food Your Way, 104
    Shrimp on a Limb, 164

side dishes, 115–40
    "Belgian" Slaw, 129
    Can't Beet This, 117
    Confetti Farfalle, 121
    Mixed Bag, 125
    Not Mean Greens, 124
    Oui, Oui, Mon Cherie!, 122
    Quinoa Tabbouleh, 126
    Rosie's Better Beans, 119
    The Tahini Thrill, 123
    Tina's Famous Farro, 134
    Wild about Veggies, 116
    Yam, Yam Good!, 138

slaws, "Belgian" Slaw, 129

sliders, Do the Salmon Slide, 81

smoothies
    Boost-My-Mood Banana Smoothie, 31
    Love Me, Love My Smoothie, 37
    Mother Nature's Green Machine, 35
    Superberry Smoothie, 25
    Take-Me-Away Tropical Fruit Smoothie, 42

snacks, 159–82
    Butternut Squash Mix 'n' Mash, 160
    Chocolate Peanut Butter Power Bites, 176
    Dynamite Egg Poppers, 169
    Flipped-Out Flapjacks, 166
    Irresistible Almond-Garlic Dip, 175
    Let's Roll, 165
    Naturally Nutritious Power Bars, 180
    Pickle My Fancy, 173

    Presto Pesto Bean Dip, 170
    Roll Model, 179
    Saucy Beef Bonbons, 174
    Scoop My Salsa, 177
    Shrimp on a Limb, 164
    A Star Is Born Popcorn, 161
    Strawberries on a Cloud, 163

snapper, 83

snow peas, 75

soups
    Beyond Belief, 92
    bouillabaisse, 104
    Perfect Pumpkin Soup, 97
    See Food Your Way, 104
    Tuscan Winter Warmer, 102

sour cream, 142

soy sauce
    Oodles of Noodles Salad, 139
    Super Simple Sensation, 84

spaghetti squash, Oh, My! Spaghetti Surprise, 67

spinach
    Green Eggs and Ham Torpedo, 33
    New Dehli Belly, 47
    Rev Up 'n' Go Baked Eggs, 24
    Spin the Wheel, 89

spreads
    Irresistible Almond-Garlic Dip, 175
    Power Pesto, 96
    Presto Pesto Bean Dip, 170
    Simply Peachy, 39

squash
    butternut squash, 97, 101, 134, 160
    Butternut Squash Mix 'n' Mash, 160
    Farmer's Harvest, 128
    Italian Rice Is Nice, 101
    Oh, My! Spaghetti Surprise, 67
    Perfect Pumpkin Soup, 97
    pumpkin, 97, 187
    Rat-a-Tat-Tat, 108
    spaghetti squash, 67

Tina's Famous Farro, 134

    yellow squash, 108, 128

stir-fry, 75

strawberries

    Keep Your Eye on the Pizza Pie, 107

    Mighty Melon-Berry Float, 156

    Strawberries on a Cloud, 163

    Tasty Trio, 58

    Tutti Fruitti, 21

strawberry preserves, 147, 149

sunflower seeds, 180

sweet potatoes

    Flipped-Out Flapjacks, 166

    Hot Mama, 78

    Irresistible Almond-Garlic Dip, 175

    Little Miss Savory Muffins, 23

sweets, Chocolate Peanut Butter Power Bites, 176

Swiss chard

    Bundles of Joy, 109

    Simply Savory Stuffed Pork, 70

    Tina's Famous Farro, 134

T

tabbouleh, Quinoa Tabbouleh, 126

tacos, Easy Breezy Island Tacos, 86

tahini

    Happy Veggie Pocket, 59

    Oodles of Noodles Salad, 139

    The Tahini Thrill, 123

tapenade, 57, 122

tarragon, 173

teas

    Creamy Dreamy Orange Tea, 188

    Earl Grey Pear Latte, 189

    Hibiscus-Ginger Refresher, 190

    "Min-Tea" Energizer, 193

tempeh, 92

thyme

    Can't Beet This, 117

    Dynamite Egg Poppers, 169

    Homemade Holiday Hit, 71

    The Lean Machine, 73

    The Meatless Mediterranean, 83

    Oh, My! Spaghetti Surprise, 67

    Rat-a-Tat-Tat, 108

    Saucy Beef Bonbons, 174

    See Food Your Way, 104

    Simply Peachy, 39

    Simply Savory Stuffed Pork, 70

    Squeeze Me!, 50

    Strawberries on a Cloud, 163

tomatoes

    Beyond Belief, 92

    Bundles of Joy, 109

    Charming Charmoula, 88

    Farmer's Harvest, 128

    Fish in Paradise, 85

    kippers, 60

    The Lean Machine, 73

    Make My Meatballs, 74

    The Marvelous Mediterranean, 113

    The Meatless Mediterranean, 83

    Oh, My! Spaghetti Surprise, 67

    Oui, Oui, Mon Cherie!, 122

    Quinoa Tabbouleh, 126

    Rev Up 'n' Go Baked Eggs, 24

    Roll Model, 179

    Rosie's Better Beans, 119

    Saucy Beef Bonbons, 174

    The Scandalous Scandinavian, 52

    Scoop My Salsa, 177

    See Food Your Way, 104

    Shrimp on a Limb, 164

    Siesta Special, 135

    Squeeze Me!, 50

    Super Simple Sensation, 84

    Tuna Tune-Up, 57

    Tuscan Winter Warmer, 102

    Velvety Veggie Mac 'n' Cheese, 98

    Zorba the Greek, 76

toppings, Raspberry Coulis, 143

tortillas, 33, 46, 58, 86

tuna, 57

turkey

    Bundles of Joy, 109

    Hot Mama, 78

turkey bacon, 179

turmeric, 109

turnips, 173

V

vegetables

    Can't Beet This, 117

    Flipped-Out Flapjacks, 166

    Happy Veggie Pocket, 59

    Pickle My Fancy, 173

    sweet potatoes, 23

    Wild about Veggies, 116

    zucchini, 23

vegetarian chili, meatless main courses, 92

Vidalia onions

    Kippers and Bits, 60

    Mixed Bag, 125

vodka

    Blueberry Cassis Fizz, 196

    Orange Vodka Snowball, 194

W

wakame, 118

walnuts

    Butternut Squash Mix 'n' Mash, 160

    Chicken Salad Sammy, 48

    Heart Throb, 136

    Tina's Famous Farro, 134

    Yummy Chunky Chocolate Brownies, 150

wasabe, 179

watermelons, 156

wheat germ, Superberry Smoothie, 25

Whey to Go Yogurt Brûlée, 148

white beans, 170

white vinegar, 173

white wine, 84, 93, 104, 116

wild mushrooms, Wild about Veggies, 116

Y

yams, 138

yellow squash

    Farmer's Harvest, 128

    Rat-a-Tat-Tat, 108

yogurt, frozen

    The Apple of My Eye, 147

    Mighty Melon-Berry Float, 156

    Orange Vodka Snowball, 194

yogurt, Greek

    Best Pesto Scramble, 43

    Happy Veggie Pocket, 59

    Little Miss Savory Muffins, 23

    Meatless Madness, 112

    Mix it Up Müesli, 18

    Mother Nature's Green Machine, 35

    New Dehli Belly, 47

    Over the Rainbow, 153

    Power Nutrient Parfait, 30

    Superberry Smoothie, 25, 31

    Whey to Go Yogurt Brûlée, 148

    Zorba the Greek, 76

Z

zucchini

    Beyond Belief, 92

    Farmer's Harvest, 128

    Hot Mama, 78

    Little Miss Savory Muffins, 23

    Pickle My Fancy, 173

Rat-a-Tat-Tat, 108

About the Author

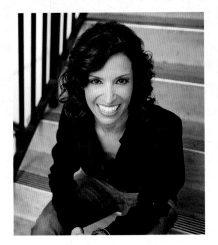

TINA RUGGIERO, M.S., R.D., L.D., is a sought-after nutrition expert, spokesperson and award-winning author. Fondly called "The Gourmet Nutritionist," Tina is frequently seen on national TV, heard on radio, and her writing, recipes and advice have appeared in magazines and newspapers, including *Men's Health*, *USA Today*, *Family*, *Woman's World* and *First for Women*. Tina is the principal of her own nutrition consulting firm where she helps both corporations and consumers. She is also a nutrition correspondent for NBC's syndicated television show *Daytime*; a special correspondent to the *Tampa Tribune* and an avid cook . Her first book, *The Best Homemade Baby Food on the Planet* was a finalist in the prestigious IACP cookbook competition. Tina's blog, found at www.tinaruggiero.com, is often cited in magazines, newspapers and on the Internet for its reliable, accurate and inspiring content. You can follower her on Twitter @Tina_Ruggiero.